Drugging Kids

Psychiatry's Wholesale Drugging of Schoolchildren for ADHD

C. L. Garrison

DRUGGING KIDS — PSYCHIATRY'S WHOLESALE
DRUGGING OF SCHOOLCHILDREN FOR ADHD

Be Awake Press, Publisher
Boston, MA, USA

Editing by Rosary Shepherd
Design by Eric Conover of All3Publishing.com

ISBN for print edition: 978-1-63443-764-6
ISBN for ebook edition: 978-1-63443-763-9

Contents

Introduction

The Need for a Healthy Skepticism

Some American psychiatrists came up with a diagnosis known as Attention Deficit Hyperactivity Disorder, commonly known as ADHD. They didn't find the disorder within their patients' bodies like typical medical diseases, but they agreed that certain common behaviors often found in children should be considered as symptoms of a mental disorder. The list of symptoms was printed in the American Psychiatric Association's *Diagnostic and Statistical Manual of Mental Disorders,* allowing them to collect insurance payments for treating millions of children.

Thus today, in America, parts of Europe and Australia, tremendous numbers of children are made to take drugs based on the assumption that they have this so-called mental disorder, ADHD. Historically, the diagnosis has been assigned to boys far more than girls, making it obvious that often normal, boyhood characteristics have been considered as symptoms of this fabricated disease.

The drugs most commonly used on children labeled as having Attention Deficit Hyperactivity Disorder are the stimulant drugs methylphenidate and various forms of amphetamines. For instance, the common ADHD drug Ritalin is comprised of the chemical methylphenidate, and Adderall is composed of several amphetamines.

A justification that has often been given for drugging children with psychiatric stimulants is that the children have defects in their brains, which are somehow made up for by "medicating" them with these substances. The problem is, these supposed brain defects have never been located, despite decades of research. When a psychiatrist tells parents that their child has a condition called Attention Deficit Hyperactivity Disorder that is being caused by a "chemical imbalance in the child's brain," the psychiatrist making this diagnosis has no physical proof for this statement which he can show the parents or anybody else. He is only offering an opinion.

Americans should realize that psychiatric and psychological treatments are often experimental. Psychiatrists cannot find the diseases and mental disorders they say they are treating and very often their treatments cause actual physical damage to the bodies of their patients.

In every decade, people tend to think that the "medical" practices of their day and age are correct and far advanced over practices of previous decades and centuries. But, since Man has been adopting this view over and over for ages, perhaps a little more skepticism about some of today's treatments would be wiser.

The lobotomy was a standard psychiatric treatment at the middle of the 20th century, in which a psychiatrist would take an instrument resembling an ice pick (or an actual ice pick in the case of the famous lobotomist and psychiatrist Walter Freeman) and drive it up through the soft tissue behind the eyeballs of a patient, where he would make slashing motions with the instrument, severing connections between the frontal lobe of the patient's brain from the rest. Though today we view this treatment as barbaric, it was an accepted psychiatric practice in America until 1965.

The "father of American psychiatry," whose face adorns the symbol of the American Psychiatric Association, was Benjamin Rush. He was a leading proponent for a medical practice in his day known as bloodletting, in which patients' veins were punctured and pints or liters of blood were drained from their bodies in the belief that it would cure them. This treatment contributed to the deaths of many people in history, including the first President of the United States, George Washington, who died after several bloodlettings in 1799 when he was being treated for a sore throat.

Lobotomies and bloodletting were widely accepted practices in their day, mainly because people who were viewed as authorities said the treatments were the right things to do. Thus, today, one can certainly have a healthy skepticism about recommendations from someone in the field of mental health, especially if they are telling you to drug your child for a disease that hasn't been found in the child's body.

There are side effects from taking ADHD drugs that will follow America's children to their graves; indeed, there are reasons to believe that the drugs are likely to hasten their arrival to their graves. However, the psychiatric drugging of children is a multi-billion dollar industry from which people from the mental health and pharmaceutical industries reap enormous financial gains.

This book will shed more light on the potential damaging effects of drugging children with psychiatric stimulant drugs, the lack of science to the diagnosis of ADHD and some of the incentives behind the widespread, psychiatric drugging of children that is occurring in the Western World today.

The chapters in the book are essentially comprised of assertions and examples of evidence supporting them. Much of the book is in the form of direct quotations excerpted from studies found in medical journals, news articles and other publications. As I have been studying about the drugging of children for so-called ADHD for several decades, some of the references cited and quotations from them were published decades ago. I have put quotations in bold type, as I believe many of them are particularly informative. Some of the quotations may contain minor, grammatical errors or misspellings, but I have taken pains not to alter them.

Where I have used quotations, I have cited the sources of these references in the text, and I have listed them all by chapter at the end of the book. Parents, or any readers, should be able to locate many of the references simply by looking them up on the internet and just typing in the title of the research study or article. Researching these articles for oneself will help the reader draw his or her own conclusions about the current widespread practice of drugging schoolchildren for ADHD. The main purpose of this work is to inform and educate people about aspects they haven't known about ADHD and its treatments.

Many of the studies cited were conducted on methylphenidate (commonly referred to as Ritalin) because there has been so much research and written material about this drug, since it has been a primary stimulant provided for ADHD for so long.

I have briefly defined some of the medical and scientific terms used in the quotations, either just before or shortly after the quotations are used.

In researching the material for this book it was apparent that ADHD and the stimulant drugs that are used to treat it are topics many people have strong feelings about, both pro and con. I am aware of the different viewpoints.

In writing this book I am not trying to deny that some students have trouble paying attention or have a tendency to be more active than others. This is obviously true. I myself would probably have been labeled ADHD had I been going to school in the 1990's or early 21st century. I was young for my class and extremely disinterested in school in my first three grades. In third grade I was sent to a guidance counselor. She was not trained in psychology particularly, as such people are today; she was an expert in teaching reading. She asked me to say the alphabet and I couldn't say it completely. I realized at that point I had better buckle down a bit on my studies and I soon caught up with my class. That was in 1955.

In those days, to my knowledge, no kids in my classes were being labeled with psychiatric diagnoses and being put on psychiatric drugs. I don't recall any students in all my classes up through high school and through college being prescribed psychiatric drugs. Our institutions of learning seemed to function relatively smoothly without them.

C. L. Garrison

2014

DRUGGING KIDS

Section I

Side Effects from ADHD Drugs No Child Would Want

Chapter One

Physical Side Effects from ADHD Drugs

There can be many short- and long-term side effects from taking psychiatric drugs. In America today, there are thousands of individuals who display permanent neurological damage from being treated with them. When you see someone walking oddly or having uncontrollable facial movements or rolling their tongue outward, the chances are you are looking at a person who was administered psychiatric drugs and whose nervous system is consequently permanently damaged.

Any psychiatric drug causes many effects to a person's body. The "side effects" are simply those that are additional to the intended effect that the drug is supposed to bring about. In the case of psychiatric drugs, none of the effects are normal. One could take a medicine that caused a normal effect, such as in the case of a diabetic taking insulin because his body wasn't producing enough of the substance on its own. However, when one is prescribed a psychiatric drug, every effect in the body is essentially abnormal.

The drugs that are most often prescribed for Attention Deficit Hyperactivity Disorder are usually from the category of drugs known as "stimulants." Sometimes they are referred to as psychostimulants. The ADHD drugs are usually comprised of the chemical methylphenidate or amphetamines. Examples of these drugs made of methylphenidate are Ritalin and Concerta. Examples of ADHD drugs made of amphetamines are Adderall, Vyvance and Dexedrine.

Some of the side effects that are commonly found in children who are put on a stimulant drug for ADHD include headaches, stomach discomfort, increased heart rate, raised blood pressure, changes in mood, loss of appetite, weight loss, difficulty falling asleep (insomnia), and suppressed body growth.

Unfortunately, psychiatrists who prescribe stimulants often play down the side effects of the drugs. Many psychiatric drugs have been marketed with a lack of emphasis on their side effects and addictive qualities, then later have been found to be both addictive and physically damaging to patients. For example, the drug Cylert, which used to be a drug commonly prescribed for children considered to be "ADD" or "hyperactive," was found to be associated with liver deterioration. It went into disfavor as a drug to prescribe and in 2005 its manufacturer, Abbott Laboratories, took it off the market.

If one looks over the information sheet that accompanies a container of an ADHD drug, one may see dozens of adverse side effects that it could cause. Many of the terms used to name the diseases that can be caused may be stated in medical terminology, making their comprehension difficult for most parents.

Growth Suppression from Ritalin and Other ADHD Drugs

"Growth suppression" has been known as a side effect from taking Ritalin and other ADHD drugs for a long time. A study titled "Effect of long-term treatment of hyperactive children with methylphenidate," published in the *Canadian Medical Association Journal* in 1975 stated:

> **Findings suggest that children who take methylphenidate even in moderate doses for several years may in some cases fail to grow at expected rates.**

Some doctors will try to ease parents' concerns about an ADHD drug stunting the growth of their children by mentioning that they can expect their children to grow at faster rates once taken off the drug. However, this is a reckless dismissal of what should be a very disturbing side effect. What's more, it is very common for children to be kept on an ADHD drug for years at a time. Worse still, some physicians try to keep patients on a drug not only through childhood, but into their adult years when their bodies have stopped growing.

Very young children are sometimes administered ADHD drugs, despite warnings from their manufacturers not to administer these drugs before the age of six. The growth damage done to children from taking a stimulant drug in these sensitive years of physical development is likely to be significant.

A forthcoming chapter in this book addresses the side effect of stunted growth from ADHD drugs in greater depth.

Serious Addiction As a Side Effect of ADHD Drugs

There is another aspect of ADHD drugs that is very important and that is that they can be very addictive, especially when they are being abused. Abusing a drug means that one is using it without a prescription or using it with a prescription in a way that it is not intended to be used, such as a patient raising his or her dose of the drug too much and too fast on their own. ADHD drugs can become so addictive that some people have tremendous difficulty coming off of the drugs because the physical and psychological withdrawal effects become too hard to bear. The effects can become especially severe if one has been taking very high doses of the drug and has not been sleeping or eating properly for prolonged periods of time.

Addiction has become an increasingly important aspect of ADHD drugs, since, in today's schools in America, they are being sold and shared widely amongst high school and college students. It has also become quite common today for students to pretend that they have ADHD symptoms so that mental health practitioners will give them prescriptions for monthly quantities of the drugs, which the students can then take in any amount they decide or distribute and sell to other students. Students who obtain ADHD drugs in these illegal ways tend to take them in unusually high doses.

A later chapter in this book addresses the matter of ADHD drug addiction in much greater detail.

Trying to Keep our Children from Being Polluted

It is common knowledge today, and a worthwhile cause, that we should be trying to safeguard our children, ourselves and future generations from environmental toxins of all sorts. We work to see that our water supplies are safe, our air is clean, that bottles of cleaning solutions are labeled if hazardous, that our processed foods are also labeled and their components described on their packaging.

Currently, teachers in many schools throughout the United States and countries across the world try to awaken their pupils to the dangers of environmental toxins. How ironic it is that before many of the students come to school in the morning they have been made to ingest drugs that are foreign substances to their bodies and have a vast array of damaging, unhealthy side effects. Even more ironic is the fact that it is often school personnel themselves who have initiated steps to get the children put on drugs, sometimes for years at a time or even the majority of their childhoods.

The current, widespread trend of drugging schoolchildren with psychiatric drugs began primarily with the "Attention Deficit" and "Hyperactivity" diagnoses in the last quarter of the twentieth century. Today, children in the Western World are often sent to school with various other psychiatric diagnoses and drugs as well. Today's classrooms may have 15 to 20 percent of their pupils taking one or more psychiatric drugs on a daily basis. This is, unfortunately, a kind of daily, direct, in-your-mouth pollution of our nation's children.

In the March 31, 2013 *New York Times* was an article titled "A.D.H.D. Seen in 11% of U.S. Children as Diagnoses Rise," by reporters Alan Schwarz and Sarah Cohen. They were reviewing statistics that had recently been put out by the federal Centers for Disease Control and Prevention (CDC). One of the data they noted was that **'About one in 10 high-school boys currently takes A.D.H.D. medication....'**

That's 10% of America's high school boys taking amphetamines or amphetamine-type drugs on a daily basis. Additionally, many of our country's high school girls are taking the same drugs.

America's schoolchildren are being exploited and have been turned into a gigantic drug market. Outlandish as the whole situation is, psychiatric marketers are still saying there are a lot more children who should be diagnosed and drugged for ADHD.

These drugs can have very serious side effects, as the next few chapters will illustrate in greater detail.

Chapter Two

ADHD Drugs and Shortening of Life Span

One could reasonably conclude that since psychiatric ADHD drugs often increase pulse rate and blood pressure, they could be expected to reduce the life span of people who have been subjected to them for several years, especially in the cases of children. This seems all the more likely when you consider other negative, physical side effects the drugs create, such as weight loss, decreased appetite, insomnia and stunted body growth. These are not phenomena a child should have occurring when his or her body is trying to develop and grow.

Even more extreme shortening of life span must occur in cases where youth start to abuse ADHD drugs by taking them recklessly, at first to cram for exams or for recreational use and later taking them in higher and higher doses as they become addicted. Unfortunately, this type of drug abuse is happening increasingly in our nation's high schools and especially in our colleges. In such cases students may get little or no sleep for several nights in a row and simultaneously eat very little food while their heart may be pumping unnaturally fast. A student may start doing this over and over again in an effort to succeed at his or her studies. As an example, the following is an excerpt from a statement a former Adderall addict had on a website (which can be found in the bibliography for this chapter at the end of the book). The passage is presented as it was written:

There would be times where I would be in a final exam, having not slept for three days and it would take me five minutes to write a single sentence. My brain literally couldn't function. Things slept from my mental grip like a wet bar - I was paranoid. I would only eat a banana a day, and I was always sleep deprived.

The individual who had this statement posted on the internet seemed to want to alert people to the dangers of abusing this drug. There are now many students who abuse ADHD drugs on a regular basis in an effort to keep their grades up or because they are addicted and have trouble facing the inevitable "crashes" that have to occur when they come down off the drugs. Students who become addicted to ADHD stimulants are very likely to be doing serious damage to their brains and bodies. Such behavior is becoming a fact of life in many of our nation's universities as ADHD stimulant drugs continue flooding into the dorms and apartments of the students, both legally and illegally.

Students who become addicted to ADHD stimulants sometimes get suicidal when they can no longer get the drugs. Occasionally, such a student will take his own life. An example of this occurring is given in a forthcoming chapter.

There have been some cases of children dying long before the end of their expected life span from taking psychiatric drugs for ADHD, even when they were not abusing the drugs and were following a doctor's orders conscientiously. In February, 2005, Health Canada temporarily banned the marketing of the ADHD drug Adderall because of a report of 20 sudden deaths associated with the drug, 14 of them being children. As it turned out from further examination, some of the children who died had other circumstances, which along with the ADHD stimulant, contributed to their passing. Apparently, a few had heart conditions or diabetes and one was also dehydrated at the time of death. None of the deaths occurred in Canada, but Canadian regulators were worried. They later lifted the ban.

According to an Associated Press story out of Pontiac, Michigan on April 17, 2000, a medical examiner said that **"long-term use of Ritalin may have led to a 14-year-old boy's death."** The article went on to state:

Matthew Smith collapsed at his home on March 21 and was pronounced dead a short time later. Oakland County Medical Examiner Ljubisa Dragovic concluded that the boy died of a heart attack likely caused by

10 years of taking Ritalin for attention deficit hyperactivity disorder. Smith's family told Dragovic Matthew occasionally complained of chest discomfort and racing heart.

In the May 8, 2000 issue of the WorldNetDaily, Dr. Dragovic was quoted as saying about Matthew's death from Ritalin:

"There was a chronic change of the heart muscle and the small blood vessels in the heart. This comes about from long-term exposure. This kid was on (Ritalin) repeatedly for 10 years."

Dragovic said that after a thorough analysis he found the boy's small blood vessels manifesting scarring and tissue growth consistent with chronic stimulant use.

On his website, ritalindeath.com, Matthew's father also tells of further damage that was caused to his son's heart from taking the ADHD drug:

I was told by one of the medical examiners that a full-grown man's heart weighs about 350 grams and that Matthew's heart's weight was about 402 grams. Dr. Dragovic said this type of heart damage is smoldering and not easily detected with the standard test done for prescription refills. The standard test usually consists of blood work,

listening to the heart, and questions about school behaviors, sleeping and eating habits.

What is important to note here is that Matthew did not have any pre-existing heart condition or defect.

An article published by MSNBC on May 2, 2000, also highlighted the danger to the heart from Ritalin:

Stephanie Hall was 11 years old when she died in her sleep. Matthew Smith was 14 when he collapsed while skateboarding. Both were taking methylphenidate, most commonly known as Ritalin, when they died of sudden heart failure.

"I do not understand why she would die from a heart arrhythmia when there is no history," said Michael Hall, Stephanie's father.

Arrhythmia means problems with a heart's rhythm; the heartbeat may be irregular, too fast or too slow.

In an article that can be found on the internet titled "Psychotropic Drugs and Failure to Warn," a mother named Vicki Dunkle tells the story of how a school psychologist recommended to Mrs. Dunkle that her 8-year-old daughter Shaina see a doctor because she had the symptoms of ADHD. The young girl was put on an antidepressant drug called Desipramine. The article states:

In 1999 I was told by the school psychologist that my 8 year old daughter

**Shaina couldn't stay focused, talked out of
turn, couldn't concentrate and had trouble
staying on task and recommended she go to
a doctor because she had all the symptoms of
attention deficit disorder.**

The article goes on to say:

**February 26, 2001 at the age of 10
years old Shaina Louise Dunkle died. Shaina
had one grand mal seizure and died within
minutes in the arms of her parents as we
watched helpless and there was absolutely
nothing we could do but watch as her life
ended. Medical examiners final report
concluded that the main cause of death was
DESIPRAMINE TOXICITY.**

Psychiatric stimulants increase pulse rate and
though children who are put on them don't usually die
within a few years, it is highly probable that the drugs
shorten life span in the long run.

Today, ads for stimulants and literature
accompanying stimulant medications carry black box
warnings about the **"Heart-related problems"** with these
drugs. A black box warning can be required by the Food
and Drug Administration for extremely dangerous side
effects. Such a warning appears in the beginning of the
literature about a drug and has a black box around it. A
typical warning about heart-related problems that can
occur with people taking ADHD stimulants lists the

following effects: **"sudden death in patients who have heart problems or heart defects, stroke and heart attack in adults, increased blood pressure and heart rate."**

As stated above, in the case of 14-year-old Matthew Smith, sudden death can apparently occur from ADHD drugs even when children have no pre-existing heart problems or conditions.

Chapter Three

Stunted Body Growth
from Taking ADHD Drugs

The side effect of stunted body growth in children put on ADHD drugs deserves extra attention because it is apparently very common. If one happens to look at the information that goes with a typical prescription medication and is able to wade through the fine print and medical terminology, one will usually see a list of the side effects observed during trial testing of the drug. Often these side effects are recorded as having happened in a minor percentage of the patients who tried the drug during the trials. For instance, one may see statements to the effect that 3 percent of patients experienced nausea or 4 percent experienced headaches. Such trials are usually fairly short-term and the side effects are made to appear inconsequential and innocent. The side effect of stunted body growth from taking methylphenidate or the amphetamines used to treat so-called ADHD is definitely <u>not</u> a minor side effect occurring in a small percentage of patients.

As we saw in Chapter One, suppression of body growth from taking Ritalin was being spoken of in the *Canadian Medical Association Journal* in 1975. It is a side effect that was noteworthy then and has been known about for decades.

Stunted body growth from taking stimulants for ADHD is an effect which deserves much greater notoriety. Psychiatrists are used to playing down the importance of the effect, reflecting perhaps the comments of representatives from drug companies that visit their offices and marketing statements uttered at drug company-sponsored conferences.

In order to really notice the side effect of stunted body growth, a different sort of drug study has to be devised and it has to be a trial prolonged over years, not just weeks or a couple of months. When such trials have been conducted, we find that the phenomenon of suppressed body growth is a major side effect occurring in the vast majority of patients. When studies have been done regarding this phenomenon, they have typically found deficits in height in children due to taking stimulants in the range of approximately 1 centimeter per year.

In 2003, a study was published in the *Journal of Pediatric Endocrinology & Metabolism* that had been conducted by Megan C. Lisska and Scott A. Rivkees from the Department of Pediatrics of the Yale University School of Medicine. Its title was "Daily Methylphenidate Use Slows the Growth of Children: A Community Based

Study." In the first sentence of the article it was pointed out that methylphenidate is also known as Ritalin. The authors of the study stated that their 'goals were to assess whether methylphenidate, as prescribed in the community setting, influences growth.'

Their findings were surprising. The researchers' conclusions stated: 'Our findings suggest that the prevalence of growth-suppressive effects of methylphenidate is greater than previously suspected.' It certainly was. They observed 68 boys and 16 girls being treated with methylphenidate by two community clinics. The longer children were on the drugs the higher the percentages of children showing stunted body growth went. After three years of treatment they found that 76% of the boys and 90% of the girls were falling behind in their body growth. The researchers found that both the boys and girls were losing about 3-4 centimeters in height over a three-year period on the drug.

All the ADHD stimulants seem to create the same sort of effect. Another study on the effects of stimulants on body growth was conducted by A. Poulton from the Department of Paediatrics at Nepean Hospital, Penrith, and C.T. Cowell from the Institute of Paediatric Endocrinology, Children's Hospital at Westmead, New South Wales, Australia. The study was published in 2003 and titled "Slowing of growth in height and weight on stimulants: A characteristic pattern." In this study 44 boys and 7 girls were treated from 6-42 months. 32 of the children were treated with dexamphetamine (commonly sold as Dexedrine) and 19 were treated with methylphenidate. To quote some of the results from the study: **'During the first 6 months on stimulant medication 44 children (86%) had a height velocity below the age-corrected mean and there was weight loss in 39 (76%)'** After three and a half years on the stimulants, the test subjects had lost approximately 2.4 centimeters in height, on average. (In this study, when the researchers noticed weight loss occurring with the children, they encouraged their parents to cut back on the use of the drugs, such as on weekends, and encouraged the parents to get the children to eat more.) Another point that was noted in this study was that 55% of the patients had a "documented indication of reduction in appetite," showing that this is also definitely not a minor side effect of ADHD stimulants.

On January 21, 2013, the findings from another ADHD drug study by Alison Poulton and other researchers was published in the *Medical Journal of Australia*. The following is a passage from a news article about the study, written by Jared Owens, titled "Ritalin linked to growth delays in adolescent boys," published on January 22, 2013, in *The Australian*, a major national newspaper in Australia:

A Sydney University study of 65 boys receiving stimulants for ADHD found those aged between 12 and 14 had significantly lower weight and body mass than untreated boys in the same age bracket. Between 14 and 16, the medicated group were shorter, slimmer and experienced delays in puberty.

The researchers were satisfied the stimulants were the cause of stunted body growth rather than ADHD itself, because of a significant link between the dosage of the medication and the degree to which growth was reduced.

The point is that when parents or guardians are raising children with drugs for so-called ADHD, whether they are using the various drugs made with methylphenidate or those comprised of amphetamines, they are very likely to be causing the children to have stunted body growth. One could just as well expect a child to suffer the same side effect if he or she were being raised on cocaine. All three of these drugs, methylphenidate, amphetamines and cocaine, are categorized together in medical literature as stimulants because they all have similar characteristics in terms of their effects on the human body.

Traditionally, stunted body growth has been looked upon as a disease, a wide-spread development in a generation of children that one would try to prevent, such as in the case of children in a Third World nation suffering from malnutrition. However, today, many psychiatrists actively cause stunted body growth to millions of American, European and Australian children year after year. They cause this disease in the name of medicine even though ADHD, the "disease" they are supposedly treating, has never been located in their patients' bodies.

Before one puts a child on a stimulant drug for ADHD, one should ask himself or herself would this child like to grow up to have a body that is a bit shorter and smaller than his or her normal body size?

Another point to keep in mind is that if one is causing a child to have a smaller overall body and smaller internal organs, is one also causing the child to have a smaller brain?

Chapter Four

Evidence of Brain Damage and Brain Shrinkage from ADHD Drugs

It should come as no great surprise that the amphetamines or amphetamine-type drugs can cause brain damage, including loss of brain tissue and brain volume. One of the amphetamines which is illegal and abused the most is known as methamphetamine, sometimes used in a form known as "crystal meth." There have been brain scan studies done on people who have been taking methamphetamine that clearly showed severe loss of brain tissue due to abusing this drug. Some areas of their brains would show tissue loss of around 10%. A phenomenon that was noted was that the brain damage from abuse of methamphetamine was similar to the brain damage caused by the disease known as Alzheimer's. Another similarity to effects from Alzheimer's was that methamphetamine addicts experienced significant memory loss. A *New York Times* article from July 20, 2004 by Sandra Blakeslee titled "This Is Your Brain on Meth: A 'Forest Fire' of Damage" discussed findings from a brain scan study of people who had been meth addicts. The addicts' brains were studied using Magnetic Resonance Imaging (MRI), a technique that allows images to be taken of the insides of a patient's body without having to cut the body open or enter it in some other way. The pictures of the addicts' brains were interpreted in the article by Dr. Paul Thompson, a brain mapping expert from U.C.L.A. The "limbic" region of the brain referred to in the article is an important section under the cerebral cortex, the outer layer covering the brain that one usually sees in brain photographs.

The limbic region, involved in drug craving, reward, mood and emotion, lost 11 percent of its tissue. "The cells are dead and gone," Dr. Thompson said. Addicts were depressed, anxious and unable to concentrate.

The brain's center for making new memories, the hippocampus, lost 8 percent of its tissue, comparable to the brain deficits in early Alzheimer's. The methamphetamine addicts fared significantly worse on memory tests than healthy people the same age.

Findings from Brain Scans Done on Children Labeled ADHD and Drugged with Stimulants

There have been many studies that used brain scans to compare the brains of people labeled as ADD and/ or hyperactive, who had been given stimulants in their childhood, with people who had not been so labeled and drugged with stimulants.

In a 1998 article, titled "The Totality of the ADD/ ADHD Fraud," a neurologist named Fred Baughman, Jr. commented on studies that show an association between the administration of psychiatric stimulants for ADHD and the phenomenon of brain shrinkage:

> **"Experts" regularly proclaim the brain scan abnormalities of ADHD. What they faintly disclose in original reports, and hardly ever mention in subsequent review articles, is that virtually all such studies have utilized ADHD subjects on chronic stimulant therapy – the only physical variable. Instead of proving that ADHD is a disease or syndrome, they have proven, several times over, that the chronic Ritalin-amphetamine exposure they advocate for millions of children, causes brain atrophy (shrinkage).**

Baughman's observation seems true when one looks over studies comparing the brains of people who have been labeled ADHD and put on stimulants and people who have not been labeled as such, nor put on stimulants. For instance, there was a study in the July, 1996 issue of the *Archives of General Psychiatry* titled "Quantitative Brain Magnetic Resonance Imaging in Attention-Deficit Hyperactivity Disorder" which showed that 56 subjects who had been labeled ADHD had a 4.7 percent smaller total cerebral volume than 55 people not so labeled.

However, it was noted that 53 of the subjects in the group with smaller brain sizes **'had been previously treated with psychostimulants.'**

Another study published in the March, 1997 issue of the journal *Neurology* was titled "Volumetric MRI analysis comparing subjects having attention-deficit hyperactivity disorder with normal controls." This research compared the brains of 15 ADHD subjects with 15 people who hadn't been labeled with ADHD (referred to as the "controls"). The researchers found that the brains of the ADHD subjects were 5 percent smaller than the brains of the non-ADHD subjects. The study also pointed out that **"All subjects with ADHD had been placed on medication"** prior to the study.

The ADHD Brain Scan Controversy

American psychiatrists seem to be aware that they are skating on thin ice regarding their ADHD diagnoses and drugging. They have been diagnosing millions of children as having ADHD and putting them on stimulant drugs, while dozens of studies using brain scans have shown that children who have been taking ADHD drugs have developed slightly smaller brains.

In the past few decades, psychiatrists have done numerous studies using brain scans of children labeled ADHD who have been on stimulant drugs and compared them to children who have not been labeled ADHD and who have not been taking stimulants. The children in the studies who had been labeled ADHD and put on stimulant drugs were found to have slightly smaller brains. The researchers of these studies seemed to consistently ignore the factor of the stimulant drugs and simply conclude that the children had smaller brains because they had ADHD, not because they had been taking drugs while their bodies were in the process of growing. This conclusion that ADHD children have smaller brains was proclaimed in speeches and articles as though it was practically a proven fact. In the field of mental health, the viewpoint that ADHD children have smaller brains implied that it was okay to go on drugging children with stimulants because the brain shrinkage they were showing was viewed as a result of their "ADHD" condition.

However, all these studies never clarified whether the children labeled ADHD had smaller brains because of their so-called ADHD condition or because they had been taking ADHD drugs while they were growing up. There were so many studies like this that it appeared that the researchers were purposely avoiding the issue, as if they feared that they might find out that their drugs were causing the children's brains to be smaller.

In 2003, a controversial article was published in *The Journal of Mind and Behavior*, Winter 2003, Volume 24, about this issue. The article was titled "Broken Brains or Flawed Studies. A Critical Review of ADHD Neuroimaging Research" by David Cohen and Jonathan Leo. The article pointed out 30 of such studies and how they all avoided the obvious research which was needed to clarify if the ADHD stimulant drugs were causing children to have smaller brains. After all, the drugs have long been known to stunt children's overall body growth.

Not long before the above article was to be published, on October 8, 2002, the National Institutes of Health (NIH) suddenly issued a press release to the broad media titled "Brain Shrinkage in ADHD Not Caused by Medications," citing a 10-year study conducted by the National Institute of Mental Health (NIMH) that supposedly showed this. This press release was seized upon by the mental health field and spread far and wide, splattered across the internet and print media. The press release had the appearance of being a preemptive, defensive move in the debate about the causes of smaller brain sizes in children labeled with ADHD. The National Institute of Mental Health reinforced its appearance of being involved in the field of marketing.

However, the National Institute of Mental Health study was analyzed carefully and found to be lacking in scientific credibility. In an article titled "An Update on ADHD Neuroimaging Research," in *The Journal of Mind and Behavior,* Spring 2004, Volume 25, David Cohen and Jonathan Leo summarized several flaws in the NIMH study that essentially prevented it from finally settling the question of whether ADHD drugs cause brain shrinkage in children.

On March 26, 2006, Pediatric Neurologist Fred Baughman stated at an FDA meeting of the Psychopharmacologic Drugs Advisory Committee that the researchers in the NIMH study **"inexplicably...failed**

to use matched controls, voiding the study." "Controls" means a group of individuals one is comparing to the group one is studying. For instance, in many drug studies to see if a drug is effective, the control group is given fake medicine consisting of sugar, while the group one is really interested in is being given actual medicine. The control group should be "matched" by similarities to the group one is actually testing for the testing results to be seen as valid.

Brain Atrophy and Brain Disintegration Associated with Stimulants

The word *atrophy* means a failure to grow or a wasting away.

The word *cortical* refers to the cortex, which is the "external layer," "the gray matter" covering the brain.

The word *cerebral* has as one of its meanings, the overall brain.

In a study published in *Psychiatry Research*, in 1986, titled "Cortical Atrophy in Young Adults With a History of Hyperactivity in Childhood," the authors of the study, Henry A. Nasrallah et al., concluded that brain shrinkage and atrophy could be associated with having been put on psychiatric stimulants during childhood. They studied the brains of 24 young males who had been treated for hyperactivity as children. They compared them to the brains of 27 young males who had no history of psychiatric illness.

The study of the 24 males who had been treated for hyperactivity began within two years of their 21st birthdays. The study stated: **'All had been given a trial of central nervous system stimulant drugs (primarily methylphenidate) during childhood.'**

One of the observations the researchers found in this study was a phenomenon known as sulcal widening, which is a widening and splitting along the grooves and furrows of the brain. ("Sulcal" refers to the sulci, the medical term for the grooves one sees on the surface of a human brain, taken from the Latin *sulcus,* meaning furrow.) They found sulcal widening occurring in fifty-eight percent (14 out of 24) of the group that had been treated with stimulant drugs, as opposed to only 3.8 percent (1 out of 27) of the control group.

The hyperactive group in this study was referred to with the phrases "adults with a history of hyperactivity" or the "HK/MBD group", meaning those who had been labeled "hyperkinetic" and/or suffering from "minimal brain dysfunction." These were the labels that were in vogue in the 1970's to describe what we call today "Attention Deficit Hyperactivity Disorder." Today, instead of saying "hyperkinetic," we say "hyperactive."

Though the researchers who conducted this study were not positive of the full implications of their findings, they stated:

The data in this study are suggestive of mild cerebral atrophy in young male adults

who had a diagnosis of HK/MBD during childhood and had received stimulant drug treatment for a period of time.

Later in the findings they stated:

Finally, since all of the HK/MBD patients had been treated with psychostimulants, cortical atrophy may be a long-term adverse effect of this treatment.

Psychiatry's Disregard for the Probable Brain Damage Being Inflicted on Millions of Children

There are dozens of studies that have been done over the past several decades indicating an association between the use of psychiatric stimulants and the prevalence of brain shrinkage. These studies are not easy to read for someone not trained in medicine, but they can be found in professional journals, as were those cited above.

The fact that psychiatrists have not released this information to the broad public or ascertained with complete certainty the causes of the brain shrinkage found in children who have been put on stimulant drugs for ADHD are omissions that amount to a sort of criminal negligence. Their failure to do so seems to imply their guilt and reluctance to confront this reality. When such a study is conducted, it needs to be done honestly with all specifics reported with integrity.

Marked Reduction of Blood Flow to the Brain From Being Given Ritalin

Probably one of the reasons that brain shrinkage shows up as a phenomenon with people who have been brought up on ADHD drugs is that these drugs apparently reduce blood flow to the brain.

Again, the word "cerebral" can be used to mean the entire brain of a person.

In the November, 1994 issue of *Life Sciences* was a study titled "Methylphenidate Decreases Regional Cerebral Blood Flow in Normal Human Subjects." The study was conducted on 5 healthy male subjects. In the introduction to the article it is pointed out that methylphenidate (Ritalin) is often administered as part of treatment for cocaine abusers and that it creates similar chemical reactions in the brain. The authors of the study wanted to see if it affected cerebral blood flows similarly to cocaine.

Like cocaine, methylphenidate was found to have a marked influence on the flows of blood in the body, increasing heart rate and blood pressure and decreasing the flow of blood to the brain. The tests showed a decrease in blood flow to the brains of all the subjects ranging between 23 to 30 percent as a result of receiving an injection of a normal dose of methylphenidate. The blood flows were tested about 5-10 minutes after injection and about a half-hour after injection. There was a consistent decrease in blood flow to the brains by 23 to 30 percent at both times, in all five subjects. This decrease in blood flow to the brain constitutes a 23 to 30 percent decrease in the amount of oxygen and nutrients going to brain cells as well as a decrease in the amount of waste and carbon dioxide being taken away from the brain cells. This factor might be compounded in some cases by the side effect of loss of appetite kids tend to have on these drugs, a factor which by itself would cause less nutrients to be going to the brain.

For a growing child's brain to have this kind of reduction in nutrients and oxygen occurring for years at a time, sometimes starting at ages below the age of six, cannot be healthy and may be one of the reasons for brain shrinkage associated with Ritalin and other ADHD drugs.

People Who Abuse Stimulants May Be Causing Themselves Brain Damage Through Lack of Sleep

One of the commonest side effects of ADHD drugs is that they can cause insomnia, an inability to fall asleep easily. Sometimes a child being given a stimulant drug for ADHD will require an additional medication just to sleep at night.

There is a growing trend in American high schools and colleges today of students taking stimulants to cram for exams, since the drugs can keep them energized without any sleep. They may not even have prescriptions for the drugs, but are able to get them from students who do have prescriptions by either paying them for the pills or just asking for them. After a night of staying up cramming, the drugs can be taken again in the morning to keep the students energized to take their exams and continue through the day. Sometimes students taking these drugs in this way get no sleep or very little sleep for several days in a row during exam periods. This sort of use of the drugs is actually a form of drug abuse.

When such students stop taking the drugs, they can suffer very unpleasant withdrawal effects that affect them physically and emotionally. It is not uncommon for some of these students to become somewhat addicted and dependent on the drugs, not only to get through exams, but to even function in school on a day to day basis. For the students who do this, but don't have prescriptions, and even for some that do, they will often find themselves upping their dosages to maintain the levels of energy and alertness they feel they need to keep up their grades.

One of the repercussions of taking stimulants to stay up night after night without getting sleep may be brain damage. On January 2, 2014, there was an article on *The Boston Globe* website, boston.com, titled "Pulling an all-nighter could damage brain, study suggests" by Deborah Kotz. The news article cited a Swedish research study, published in the medical journal *Sleep,* in which researchers found evidence of brain damage from the simple act of losing a single night's sleep. According to the news article the brain damage may be occurring because **'the brain is unable to flush out its toxins when forced to be in a continuous state of alertness.'**

In any case, it is quite obvious to almost anyone that sleep is very necessary and has a rejuvenating effect that makes one feel revitalized physically and mentally.

Causing Body and Brain Damage Nothing New with Psychiatry

One should not be too surprised that a routine psychiatric treatment would cause body and brain damage. Up until 1965, a standard psychiatric practice was to slice the connections of the frontal lobe of the brain to the rest of it, when performing the practice known as the prefrontal lobotomy. Electroshock, still used today, causes brain damage. Some psychiatric drugs commonly given to mental patients often cause brain shrinkage and permanent brain and nerve damage, causing patients to have uncontrollable body movements for the remainder of their lives. Indeed, causing permanent brain and nerve damage could be said to be a common denominator to many of psychiatry's treatments, including, apparently, those currently being administered to millions of today's schoolchildren.

Chapter Five

Damaging Psychological Effects from Being Diagnosed and Drugged for ADHD

Aside from the adverse physical effects that can be caused from consuming stimulants, there are a host of adverse psychological effects as well. *The International Journal of the Addictions*, published in 1986, listed 105 hazardous effects from Ritalin, taken from a review of thirty different studies and references, and the vast majority of these side effects were psychological in nature. Among the adverse effects listed were delusions, psychosis, hallucinations, aggressiveness, anxiety, severe depression and drug addiction.

The American Psychiatric Association's own *Diagnostic and Statistical Manual of Mental Disorders* has listed mental disorders having to do with amphetamine dependence and abuse. Associated features of the disorders can include depression, having paranoid ideas, irritability and social isolation.

Methylphenidate and Amphetamines Were Used to Create Psychosis During Psychiatric Experimentation on Patients

On November 15, 1998, *The Boston Sunday Globe* began publishing a four-part series of articles titled "Doing Harm: Research on the Mentally Ill," by authors Robert Whitacker and Delores Kong about experiments American psychiatrists had been conducting between the years 1973 and 1997 in which they purposely drove patients insane with the administration of psychiatric stimulants. Supposedly, the purpose of these experiments was to learn more about psychosis. The initial article listed hospitals and universities across the country that were involved in the experimentation.

According to the chart that accompanied that initial article in *The Boston Sunday Globe* of November 15, 1998, the two types of drugs that were used most to cause psychosis were amphetamines and methylphenidate. Methylphenidate was used the most.

Details of this experimentation on unwitting patients were exposed in the four-part series in the newspaper. (The writers of this series received the prestigious George Polk Award for Medical Reporting for 1998.) For the purposes of this book, two points were made very clear from the article: Methylphenidate and amphetamines can induce psychosis, and psychiatrists tend to be willing to experiment on unwitting subjects, even at the risk of causing them immense suffering and permanent psychological damage. The patients were "unwitting" because they did not really know what they were in for when they signed releases to be part of the experiments. As a profession, psychiatrists have a long history of conducting experiments on unwitting and unwilling patients.

Psychosis As an Effect of the Administration of Ritalin

CIBA-Geigy Pharmaceutical Company, the past manufacturer of Ritalin (until they merged with Sandoz to form the very large pharmaceutical corporation Novartis), published the following warnings about Ritalin:

Ritalin should be given cautiously to emotionally unstable patients such as those with a history of drug dependence or alcoholism, because such patients may increase dosage on their own initiative.

Chronically abusive use can lead to marked tolerance and psychic dependence with varying degrees of abnormal behavior. Frank psychotic episodes can occur, especially with parental abuse.

As can be seen from the above quotes by CIBA, the drug can bring out psychotic tendencies in some children if the drug is not taken as prescribed or according to doctors' orders.

Even murderous, as well as suicidal behavior have been brought forth from children on this drug. One of the most well known cases of murderous behavior associated with the administration of Ritalin was the case of a Massachusetts teenager named Ron Matthews, who killed a fellow classmate with a baseball bat.

Another Massachusetts youth named Gerard McCra shot to death his own parents and sister when he was fifteen years old. He had been on Ritalin from the age of six.

On May 20, 1999, one month after the Columbine High School massacre in Littleton, Colorado, there was a nationwide story about a boy named T. J. Soloman from a high school in Conyers, Georgia who had been taking Ritalin. He shot six of his classmates, only wounding them.

Suicidal Behavior Associated with Ritalin and Amphetamines Especially During Drug Withdrawal

The common ADHD drug Ritalin, and amphetamines, such as Adderall and Dexedrine, are highly addictive. Severe depression and suicidal behavior may result from withdrawal from these drugs.

Thus, any parent who is having their child withdrawn from Ritalin or another stimulant drug should do so under the supervision of a competent medical doctor, preferably one who is not going to put the child on another psychiatric drug as a replacement. Both the parents and the doctor should be aware that when a child first withdraws from the stimulant, his behavior may become extreme for a short while, due to the withdrawal effects all by themselves. These withdrawal effects, which may include acute depression, should eventually subside on their own as the child returns to normal.

The Effect on a Child of Telling Him He Has an Abnormal, Defective Brain and Has to Take Drugs

One of the effects of diagnosing a child as having Attention Deficit Hyperactivity Disorder is to give the child the idea that something is wrong with him and his brain. This is a very destructive thought to impose on a child, especially when there isn't any proof that it is so.

In the process of getting a child drugged for ADHD, the parents of the child have also got to be convinced that something is anatomically amiss with their child. The child's teachers and other people in their lives may also be given the same idea. These people may then seem to confirm to a child that he possesses a malfunctioning brain and that he isn't quite as good or able as others not labeled with this phantom disease.

In the American psychiatrists' marketing efforts to receive expanded insurance coverage known as "mental health parity" (equality to usual medical insurance coverage) there was a campaign to complain about the stigmatization and consequent discrimination against the mentally ill, yet such stigmatization is created for millions of American children by psychiatrists themselves through the use of their deceptive diagnoses and labels that they impose upon children with no actual proof that there is anything medically wrong with the children in the first place.

In order to market their diagnoses and labeling of children with so-called "mental disorders," psychiatrists have invented phrases to describe the supposed brain abnormalities the children are said to have. For instance, in the 1970's it was fashionable to label children as having "Minimal Brain Dysfunction."

For years, another marketing trick that was popular with psychiatrists was to tell parents that their children had "chemical imbalances in their brains" causing them to need ADHD drugs. This phrase has conveniently provided justification for drugging millions of children in America. The irony in this case is that there is no real proof of a chemical imbalance in a child's brain when the child is diagnosed as having ADHD, but as soon as a psychiatric stimulant drug is administered to the child, all manner of real chemical imbalances can be seen to occur in the child's brain and body.

Chapter Six

Drug Addiction from Taking Ritalin, Amphetamines and Cocaine and Why They Are Categorized Together

There are five categories of drugs that the Drug Enforcement Administration (D.E.A.) uses. The most dangerous and of no medical use are the Schedule I substances. The next most dangerous category is Schedule II, which is comprised of those drugs that are seen to be of some medical use, but are also viewed as highly addictive and subject to abuse. The word "abuse" here means to take a prescription drug without a prescription or take more of it than is prescribed or take it for other purposes than it is supposed to be used for. Ritalin, amphetamines and cocaine are all categorized by the D.E.A. as being Schedule II drugs. Thus their manufacture is monitored closely by the Drug Enforcement Administration.

Methylphenidate (Ritalin), amphetamines and cocaine have long been categorized together in scientific literature, mainly because they can all produce similar effects on users. To some observers their effects are virtually indistinguishable. In an article titled "Stimulant Abuse in Man," published in 1977, the authors Everett Ellinwood and Marilyne Kilbey categorized these stimulants together:

Perhaps the best-known effect of chronic stimulant administration is psychosis. Psychosis has been associated with chronic use of several stimulants; e.g., d-amphetamine and l-amphetamine, methylphenidate, phenmetrazine, and cocaine.

One of the reasons users or addicts of these drugs can become psychotic is that the drugs can keep the users awake night after night as well as diminish their appetites. Ordinarily, the human body rejuvenates itself when it sleeps, but for someone abusing these stimulants continuously, the lack of sleep and nutrition and the presence of other side effects take their toll on the person's health and sanity.

In the *Diagnostic and Statistical Manual of Mental Disorders III R,* published by the American Psychiatric Association in 1987, the authors of the manual categorized the amphetamines, including methamphetamine, and methylphenidate together:

This group includes all of the substances...such as amphetamine, dextroamphetamine and methamphetamine ("Speed"), and those with structures...that have amphetamine-like action, such as

**methylphenidate and some substances used
as appetite suppressants ("diet pills").**

The manual went on to say how similar the patterns
of use, abuse and associated features of the above
substances are to those of cocaine abuse and dependence,
as they are all "**potent central nervous system stimulants
with similar psychoactive ...effects.**"

Ritalin and Amphetamines Have
Long Histories As Street Drugs

Ritalin and amphetamines seem to have an appeal
to certain illicit-drug users who will abuse them and may
be found indulging in criminal activities as well. Both
are drugs that have long histories as illegal substances
that have been sold on the streets by drug dealers, as
well as in schools by the very students they have been
prescribed for. As common street drugs that are addictive
and subject to heavy abuse, an increase in crime has been
associated with their use. For instance, an article titled "A
prescribed urban nightmare — How two obscure, legal
drugs unleashed a wave of crime in the streets" appeared
in the February 2, 1987 issue of the Canadian weekly news
magazine *Western Report*. It described a major crime
wave in Canada's western cities that was occurring at the
hands of drug addicts who were fond of mixing Ritalin
and another prescription drug, Talwin:

**They are inexpensive pharmaceuticals,
Ritalin an amphetamine, Talwin a pain-**

killer, and they are the drugs of choice in the downtown core of each major western Canadian city. They are sold together as packages known as T&Rs; abused simultaneously, they offset each other's unpleasant side effects. The number of regular users is low, between 1000 and 3000 in each city; and the traffic is almost always confined to a single shabby district. Nonetheless, law enforcers agree, that T&Rs are responsible for more street crime than any other drugs used in the West today.

The article continued, going into greater detail with interviews with law enforcement officials from several Canadian cities.

ADHD Drugs As Illicit Drugs Sold in High Schools and on College Campuses

Since drugs like Ritalin and Adderall are so abundantly prescribed for ADHD, they are often given or sold by students to their classmates to get high on. They are also often shared or sold amongst students to boost their levels of concentration in preparation for their exams.

The practice of students selling their ADHD drugs to their classmates is very common in American high schools and colleges today.

Sixteen years ago, the Feb 12, 1998 *Boston Globe* carried an article titled "On campus, Ritalin getting attention as a good 'buzz,'" by Richard Chacon, about the illicit use of Ritalin among college students:

Some students swallow the pills, which come in tablets of 5 to 20 milligrams. But many people – especially those who take it without prescription – crush the tablets with the flat side of a knife and snort the powder.

On May 2, 2014, *The Boston Globe* ran an article by reporter Deborah Kotz titled "1 in 5 students at an Ivy League college abuse stimulant drugs." The article stated:

Even more disturbing: Nearly one in five students at an Ivy League college (that the researchers declined to identify) reported misusing a prescription stimulant – like Ritalin or Adderall used to treat attention deficit hyperactivity disorder – while studying or finishing a paper.

Apparently, some of the students abusing the drugs did not take the drugs often, while others were using the stimulants as study aids on a more repeated basis. In addition to all the students abusing ADHD drugs at the Ivy League college, there were, of course, all the students who were taking stimulants as prescribed, trying to follow their doctor's orders.

Our nation's grade schools, high schools and colleges are awash in prescription drugs. Many students get them from other students who have prescriptions, or they get them by going to a doctor and pretending to have the symptoms of ADHD. The drugs can be used to boost energy and concentration when cramming for exams, or taken for recreational use to get "high" with at parties.

One indicator of the abuse occurring with the stimulant drugs used for ADHD has been the rising numbers of young adults being admitted to emergency rooms across the country due to overdosing on the drugs themselves or in combination with alcohol. An article from *The New York Times* on August 8, 2013, titled "New Sign of Stimulants' Toll on Young" written by Sabrina Tavernise discusses this phenomenon:

> **The number of young adults who end up in the emergency room after taking Adderall, Ritalin or other such stimulants has quadrupled in recent years, federal health officials said Thursday, fresh evidence of the unexpected consequences that can result from the wide use of medicines for conditions like attention deficit disorder.**

There was an article in the June 21, 2010 *Huffington Post* titled "Adderall: The Most Abused Prescription Drug in America." The first paragraph of the article stated: **'Adderall is abused mostly by college students and young adults. Estimates are that somewhere between 20-30 percent of college students regularly abuse**

Adderall.' A college student calling himself Cguy posted the following comment regarding the article:

> **Adderall is a serious problem. I have friends who have three prescriptions, yet still have to buy off the black market. I also know of doctors who admittedly prescribe over 2000 students to Adderall (this includes Adderall XR & Vyvance). This means that one doctor alone sends 2000+ patients to the pharmacy each month to stock up on amphetamines.**

Parents of Children on ADHD Drugs Can Become Addicted to Their Children's Medications

Parents of children who have been prescribed ADHD drugs sometimes start taking their children's medications for themselves. Thus, they can become regular users and become addicted. On June 26, 2012, there was a news story on ABC NEWS by Dan Harris and Lana Zak having to do with the rise in Adderall prescriptions for woman between the ages of 26 and 39. The title of the presentation was "Supermom's Secret Addiction: Stepping Out of Adderall's Shadow." The following excerpt is a newscaster's comments about a mother named Betsy Degree who became addicted to her own son's ADHD medication:

> **Several years ago, one of Degrees's children was prescribed Adderall, a central**

nervous system stimulant, for ADHD. In a moment of desperation she stole a pill from her own child and the addiction was almost immediate.

In the news story Ms. Degree described how she began to trick the doctor who wrote her son's prescriptions to elevate the dosages and write more prescriptions. Eventually, when she couldn't get the drugs she needed from the doctor she turned to methamphetamine.

Students Can Become Addicted to ADHD Stimulants

As an example of a student who began taking an ADHD drug in high school to cram for exams and subsequently became addicted, the following is a statement by a young lady who wrote this testimony about "study drugs" when she was a sophomore in college. It was posted on NYTimes.com on June 10, 2012. She stated that she was 18 years old and from Sarasota, Florida:

I knew (and still know) that they do more harm than good, as my moods can change on a dime and my memory is worse and worse, but getting a decent grade on a test that others seem to effortlessly ace seems worth it. Adderall hasn't become a study drug to me, it's become a way of life.

Sometimes students get so severely addicted to the stimulants they initially started taking to improve their focus on their studies that disasters occur. An example of such a student who became addicted was described in detail in the Feb 2, 2013 *New York Times* news story "Drowned in a Stream of Prescriptions" by Alan Schwarz. This is an amazing article about a real occurrence. It was written about a young man named Richard Fee who was **'an athletic, personable college class president and aspiring medical student....'**

There is a passage in the article about the psychiatric facility where Richard used to get his prescriptions and the eventual toll it took on him:

It was where, after becoming violently delusional and spending a week in a psychiatric hospital in 2011, Richard met with his doctor and received prescriptions for 90 more days of Adderall. He hanged himself in his bedroom closet two weeks after they expired.

The whole article is worth reading in its entirety. It is eye-opening.

Warning

There are serious withdrawal effects that can occur when one is trying to come off of an ADHD drug. The difficulty in going through the withdrawal process varies from person to person. Generally, how difficult it is is proportional to how high the doses are one has been taking and how long one has been using the drug. If one has been abusing it and is strongly addicted, it could, of course, be more difficult.

When one stops taking an addictive ADHD stimulant, one is liable to confuse the withdrawal effects with how they will actually feel when they have fully come off the drug. When they persist and gradually recover, they should feel much better than during the beginning stages of going through the withdrawal.

The types of things one is likely to feel during withdrawal from an ADHD drug are depression, feeling tired and having low energy, anxiety, irritability and even suicidal thoughts. One may find oneself sleeping for long periods and feeling like eating a lot. The withdrawal period may last for a few weeks or even months.

If one tapers down the drug dosages gradually the withdrawal effects will be less intense.

It is recommended that one consult with a doctor to assist during the withdrawal process. It preferably would be a doctor who is not going to try to put one on another addictive drug as a solution. Another point to keep in mind is that nowadays many doctors receive free gifts and sizeable financial inducements from drug companies for selling a lot of the companies' drugs, so a doctor may have an extra vested interest in having his or her patients continually getting prescriptions for certain pills or capsules.

Conclusion

Ritalin, amphetamines and cocaine are appropriately categorized together in scientific and medical literature due to their similar effects on a user. They are appropriately categorized as Schedule II drugs by the Drug Enforcement Administration due to their likelihood of being abused and their addictive qualities.

The fact that Ritalin and amphetamines are referred to as "medications" does not change the fact that they are drugs that are addictive and subject to widespread abuse by not only street addicts, but also a vast and growing number of American students in our grade schools, high schools and colleges.

Now, many of the graduates of recent years who have grown up abusing addictive ADHD stimulants are in our workplaces and some are still addicted, still depending on stimulants to maintain an appearance of capability and normalcy. The percentages of such individuals is likely to be on the rise unless we change our course as a culture with regard to this phenomenon.

Section II

The Diagnosis of ADHD by Opinion, Not Scientific or Medical Testing

Chapter Seven

Psychiatry's *Diagnostic and Statistical Manual of Mental Disorders* and the ADHD Diagnosis

One reason this book contains a chapter about the *Diagnostic and Statistical Manual of Mental Disorders* is that the classifying of a set of common childhood behaviors and calling them a mental disorder called Attention Deficit Hyperactivity Disorder (ADHD) and publishing them in the manual has enabled a large portion of American youth to be put on addictive, physically-damaging drugs, sometimes for many years at a time.

Yet, the diagnosis, ADHD, is without solid medical or scientific foundation.

The *Diagnostic and Statistical Manual of Mental Disorders* is likewise without solid medical or scientific foundation.

These two points will become increasingly evident as one reads forward in the chapters to come.

The Manual Itself

The *Diagnostic and Statistical Manual of Mental Disorders* is a book published by the American Psychiatric Association. It is often known as the "DSM." It lists the names of supposed mental disorders and their supposed symptoms. Each "mental disorder" is assigned a number, which is referred to when applying for health insurance coverage for its treatment.

The DSM is sometimes referred to as psychiatry's insurance bible, as its main purpose is to enable mental health practitioners to obtain insurance payments for "treating" their patients for the "mental disorders" listed in the book. Treating patients in the field of psychiatry usually means getting them to start taking one or more psychiatric drugs and coming back for prescription refills month after month.

For behaviors to qualify as official mental disorders to be written into the manual, they have only had to be considered by committees of psychiatrists and approved to be in the book, but they have not had to be discovered as abnormalities in the bodies of patients, as in the case of actual medical illnesses.

When the mental disorders are diagnosed on patients, the diagnoses are not based on any medical testing of the patients' bodies, such as with blood tests, urine analyses, tissue samples or x-rays. Instead "mental disorders" are labels assigned to patients based on opinions, rather than physical evidence in the patients' bodies. If the name of the mental disorder being assigned to a patient can be found in the DSM, the chances are the psychiatrist assigning the label to the patient can collect insurance for performing a treatment for it.

The manual is now in its fifth edition, otherwise known as "DSM V." Each new edition has seen widespread revision over its predecessor as well as the addition of many new mental disorders.

The "mental disorder" described as "Attention-deficit Disorder with or without Hyperactivity" made it into the third version of the book, known as DSM III, in 1980. A revision of this manual was issued in 1987, known as the DSM IIIR. In this version of the manual, the mental disorder was condensed to "Attention-deficit Hyperactivity Disorder" or ADHD.

An Example of How Unscientific the Creating of "Mental Disorders" Can Be

Since the mental disorders in the manual cannot be located in peoples' bodies, there has been much debating over what to classify as a disorder. For instance, according to the book *Making Us Crazy*, by Herb Kutchins and Stuart A. Kirk published in 1997, when the first version of the manual was published in 1952, homosexuality was considered behavior that should be diagnosed and treated as a mental disorder. However, in the early 1970's gay activists held protests at the American Psychiatric Association's (APA) annual conventions about their lifestyle being characterized as symptomatic of a mental disorder. As the subject became more and more of an issue it became known to the APA that many of its own members were homosexuals themselves. Eventually, in late 1973, homosexuality was reclassified by the APA as no longer a mental disorder, but rather as just another "form of sexual behavior."

From the above example, we can clearly see that the classification of homosexuality as a mental disorder was never based on science. The classification was an arbitrary decision based on opinion and probably a good deal of prejudice. It was also an arbitrary decision based on opinion when homosexuality was unclassified as a mental disorder. Science simply never had anything to do with the situation either way.

And so it is with other "mental disorders" that have been dreamed up by psychiatrists in drafting their *Diagnostic and Statistical Manual of Mental Disorders.*

Problems with Reliability of the Manual

With each new revision of the manual, the American Psychiatric Association has hoped to increase the reliability and consistency of diagnoses by different psychiatrists on their various patients. The manual lists out the behavioral symptoms that one is supposed to observe for each mental disorder. It has been hoped by the authors of the manuals that the descriptions of mental disorders and their symptoms would be so accurate and precise that they would enable different psychiatrists to look at a patient's behavior and arrive at the same diagnosis and that this could occur consistently patient after patient. However, with each new revision of the manual these hopes for reliability and consistency have failed to be realized.

In their book *Making Us Crazy*, professors Herb Kutchins and Stuart A. Kirk described a study that was conducted to test the reliability of diagnosing from using the fourth edition of the manual. Though the testing of the reliability of the manual was made easier to pass than it could have been, it still yielded poor test results:

So even with this liberal definition of agreement, reliability using DSM is not particularly good. Mental health clinicians independently interviewing the same person in the community are as likely to agree as disagree that the person has a mental disorder and are as likely to agree as disagree on which of the over 300 DSM disorders is present.

Twenty years after the reliability problem became the central scientific focus of DSM, there is still not a single major study showing that DSM (any version) is routinely used with high reliability by regular mental health clinicians. Nor is there any credible evidence that any version of the manual has greatly increased its reliability beyond the previous version. The DSM revolution in reliability has been a revolution in rhetoric, not in reality.

Even if there was a consensus that could be achieved as to what "disorder" to assign to a set of "symptoms," as displayed in a person's behavior, there would still be no proof of any defect being found in the individual's body, brain or nervous system, like one would find in an actual medical diagnosis. Instead, the psychiatric diagnosis would be based purely on opinion.

Attention Deficit Hyperactivity Disorder

This "disorder" has paid off handsomely for many mental health and pharmaceutical concerns. Again this "disorder" is diagnosed not by finding anything really wrong with a "patient's" brain, nervous system or body; indeed, the *Diagnostic and Statistical Manual of Mental Disorders* has even stated directly **"There are no laboratory tests that have been established as diagnostic in the clinical assessment of Attention-Deficit/ Hyperactivity Disorder."** Instead, it has sometimes been initially "diagnosed" by a teacher or parent checking off certain characteristics from a checklist, based on a set of criteria devised by the authors of the diagnostic manual.

According to the manual, in order to do an ADHD diagnosis on a child, a doctor is supposed to find that the child has 6 out of the supposed 9 symptoms for "Inattention," and he's supposed to find that the child has had these behaviors for at least the past 6 months. Similarly, the child can be diagnosed as having ADHD if he has 6 out of 9 supposed symptoms of "Hyperactivity and Impulsivity," and has had them for the past 6 months.

According to the manual, other conditions for the diagnosis are supposed to be met as well.

One will notice that often the behaviors listed as symptomatic of supposed ADHD seem like everyday, normal childhood actions. For example, the list of possible symptoms that are supposedly criteria for diagnosing a child as having ADHD starts off with **"Often fails to give close attention to details or makes careless mistakes in schoolwork, at work, or with other activities."**

Another diagnostic criteria for ADHD is **"Often avoids, dislikes, or is reluctant to do tasks that require mental effort over a long period of time (such as schoolwork or homework)."**

Let's look at this. Did you ever know any kid who "disliked" having to do homework? If this has been the case for over six months the child has one of the criteria for ADHD.

As many of America's teachers have been made into a nationwide referral network for the mental health industry, through required psychology courses in their college training and yearly continuing education programs, it has often been teachers who began the process of getting some of their own students drugged by checking off a few of the behavior characteristics that supposedly indicate that a child has ADHD.

But checkmarks on a list, whether from a teacher or a parent, do not constitute the presence of a real disease. As child neurologist Dr. Fred Baughman points out in

64

his article "Immunize Your Child Against Attention Deficit Disorder (ADD)": **'How could this be? How can a behavioral checklist or any paper-pencil test prove the presence of a brain disease. The answer is that none can. Not ever!'**

The DSM criteria for the diagnosing of ADHD might sound a bit complex and time-consuming for a diagnosis. But realize that in the everyday world of mass diagnosing of children, teenagers and college students, all these criteria are sometimes hardly looked at and analyzed by the psychiatrist or doctor doing the supposed diagnosis. Instead, often a quick conversation can be had with a parent about their child, or a high school or college student can say he is having difficulty concentrating on his schoolwork, and a prescription can be written for a month's supply of an amphetamine, and refills can be prescribed month after month, and year after year, as long as the "patient" and psychiatrist both want to perpetuate the arrangement.

The Diagnostic Manual Fits Psychiatry

The *Diagnostic and Statistical Manual of Mental Disorders* is a fitting part of the overall field of psychiatry. Psychiatrists pose as being in the field of medicine though they cannot locate the supposed diseases they are treating in the bodies of their patients and they list their unlocatable mental disorders in this manual that looks like a regular doctor's book of actual, physical diseases.

Furthermore, in addition to the *Diagnostic and Statistical Manual of Mental Disorders* being a pretense of being a real medical manual of diseases, many psychiatrists don't even pretend to use the pretense! Instead, they may talk to a student or parent for a few minutes and issue a prescription on the spot.

The process of college students getting addictive, ADHD drugs through some college infirmaries has been unusually easy and careless for many university students. It is quite common today for American high school and college students to fake having ADHD symptoms in order to get prescriptions for drugs so they can pull all-nighters cramming for exams or get high with the drugs or sell their pills to other students. Since there are no medical tests for an ADHD diagnosis, the students can pretend to be distracted or just tell the mental health practitioner that they are having trouble concentrating or have anxiety, and that might be enough to walk away with a prescription.

The point is, the diagnosing process for ADHD and other mental "disorders" is so loose and unscientific, it is easily taken advantage of by both patients and psychiatrists.

The *Diagnostic and Statistical Manual* is the Keystone That Holds the Whole Charade Together

As ridiculous as the mental disorders listed in the DSM may seem and even though there is no way to find these disorders in patients' bodies and even though diagnoses of the disorders are done by mere opinions, this book has become an agreed-upon device upon which a great deal of economic activity depends. Psychiatrists, psychologists, doctors, psychiatric drug manufacturers and medical insurance providers all depend on this book as a sort of catalyst that permits their economic transactions to occur. And many of them know how ridiculous the disorders are. Some psychiatrists who diagnose patients for ADHD hardly bother to refer to the statements in the DSM about how to do the diagnosis. The diagnosis of ADHD has gotten so casual it is often done within a short conversation during a patient's first meeting with a psychiatrist.

The DSM is the keystone for the whole charade.

The next two chapters provide further illustration of how unscientific and non-medical the diagnosing of so-called ADHD is, and consequently how dangerous and expensive it can get for society.

Chapter Eight

The Younger Students in Classrooms Tend to Be Diagnosed ADHD Considerably More Than the Older Ones

This chapter presents examples of the ADHD diagnosis having been assigned to children because they were behaving the way children at their ages normally behave.

In almost all classrooms, there is an age spectrum of the students in the room. In other words, a classroom of children around five years old may have kids who have just turned five in the past month combined with other children who are about to turn six years old. You may find some classrooms with children with year-and-a-half differences in age. For example, you could find classrooms with children ranging between early-five-year-olds up through the age of six-and-a-half-year-olds. The maturity levels of these two ends of the age spectrum are likely to be very different, as the six-and-a-half-year-old has lived about 30 percent longer than the child who just turned five.

According to an article published on the blog known as *The Well* on November 20, 2012, titled "Younger Students More Likely to Get A.D.H.D. Drugs," by reporter Anahad O'Connor, a recent study found that younger children in a grade tended to be labeled ADHD more than the older students in the same grade:

The new study found that the lower the grade, the greater the disparity. For children in fourth grade, the researchers found that those in the youngest third of their class had an 80 to 90 percent increased risk of scoring in the lowest decile on standardized tests. They were also 50 percent more likely than the oldest third of their classmates to be prescribed stimulants for A.D.H.D.

This study was based on observation of data concerning over 10,000 students in Iceland and was published in the journal *Pediatrics*.

Other studies have been showing the same phenomena occurring in schools in Canada and the United States.

According to a news story of March 6, 2012, on the website psychcentral.com titled "Youngest Kids in Class Get More ADHD Diagnoses, Drugs," younger children in the Canadian province of British Columbia have also been the students most targeted for ADHD drugging. A study involving 937,943 children went on for 11 years between December 1, 1997 and November 30, 2008. The article states:

A new Canadian study finds that the youngest children in a classroom are significantly more likely to be diagnosed with attention-deficit/hyperactivity disorder (ADHD) than their peers in the same grade.

Later in the article it stated:

Researchers found that children were 39 percent more likely to be diagnosed and 48 percent more likely to be treated with medication for ADHD if born in December compared to January.

Since this study involved observing data concerning approximately a million school children, one can infer that some tens of thousands of them were being diagnosed as having ADHD and put on drugs, mainly because they were acting like kids normally do at their age. The characteristics of this normal, age-appropriate behavior were being viewed as symptoms of ADHD because the kids were acting immaturely compared to the older students in their classrooms. Since there are no medical tests for ADHD, probably many thousands of these children were then "diagnosed" by arbitrary opinion and many of them put on stimulant drugs, with all of their side effects, such as those mentioned in the article: **'sleep disruption, increased risk of cardiovascular events and slower growth rates.'**

Other studies concerning the same phenomenon occurring in the United States have come out in the last few years. One of those U.S. studies was conducted at Michigan State University. It was published on the website for the university, MSU NEWS, on Aug. 17, 2010. The title of the article is "Nearly 1 million children potentially misdiagnosed with ADHD, study finds." The article concerned research done by a Michigan State economist named Todd Elder. It stated:

According to Elder's study, the youngest kindergartners were 60 percent more likely to be diagnosed with ADHD than the oldest children in the same grade. Similarly, when that group of classmates reached the fifth and eighth grades, the youngest were more than twice as likely to be prescribed stimulants.

Overall, the study found that about 20 percent - or 900,000 - of the 4.5 million children currently identified as having ADHD likely have been misdiagnosed.

So one can see by the above examples that the diagnosing process for ADHD is obviously very arbitrary and unscientific because there are no real, validating medical tests for the supposed disorder. This lack of science and medical testing in the diagnosing process has already lead to a great number of children worldwide being labeled and drugged for ADHD simply because they were among the youngest in their classrooms when they started going to school.

This unscientific diagnosing has, of course, cost taxpayers and people paying monthly medical insurance bills millions, if not billions, of dollars in wasted and destructive expenses. For most adult citizens, they have had their earnings taken away from them in both ways: as taxpayers and as health insurance purchasers.

Furthermore, tens of thousands of children must have been made to take ADHD drugs as a result of these ridiculous misdiagnoses and made to suffer numerous, unhealthy side effects, both physically and mentally.

Chapter Nine

Boyhood Characteristics Have Been Turned into Symptoms of Imagined ADHD

For a long time, one of the most obvious evidences that the ADHD diagnosis was not credible was the fact that boys were being diagnosed and labeled ADHD so much more than girls. It was as if the characteristics of being a typical boy had been made into the symptoms of a new disease. And that is actually what occurred. The new, created disease was being made to seem real by being taught about in teacher colleges and medical schools and in continuing education seminars year after year. But the fact that it was almost always boys who were being found to have ADHD made the diagnosis suspect. It was a glaring illogic, especially because it is such common knowledge that boys tend to be more active and rambunctious than girls. Furthermore, when grownups try to corral and control them, some boys will revolt or fight back to try to maintain their self-determinism. These tendencies have also made them a target for drugging.

Twenty to thirty years ago, the ratio of boys labeled ADHD to girls was about 9 boys to each girl. This ratio was recently cited on the website psychiatrictimes.com in an article titled "Neuropsychiatric Differences Between Boys and Girls With ADHD" by E. Mark Mahone, Ph.D: **'In the 1990s, the male to female ratio for ADHD was estimated to be about 9 to 1 in clinical settings....'**

In the December, 1996 issue of the magazine *Good Housekeeping*, in an article titled "The Pill That Teachers Push," the author, Jeanie Russell, stated: **'In 1990, 900,000 kids were on Ritalin. Today an astounding 2.5 million are - and some 80 percent of those are boys.'**

Gradually, in the last 25 years or so, more and more girls have been being diagnosed with ADHD. The ADHD drug industry, like many fields of business, is always compelled to expand its sales and this is done by expanding its markets. Young girls were a natural market and there are currently all manner of articles on the internet about reasons why more girls should be diagnosed ADHD and why they have been so overlooked as a market in the past. Another market for ADHD drugs which has been heavily created over the past few years is the market of "adults with ADHD." Having a greater proportion of girls labeled ADHD has helped make the diagnosis appear more legitimate.

Statistics from 2011 showed that boys were still being diagnosed ADHD about 2 and a half times as much as girls. According to a website for the Centers for Disease Control and Prevention (CDC), from a survey conducted in 2011: **"Boys (13.2%) were more likely than girls (5.6%) to have ever been diagnosed with ADHD."**

According to an article in the March 31, 2013 *New York Times,* by Alan Schwarz and Sarah Cohen, titled "A.D.H.D. Seen in 11% of U.S. Children as Diagnoses Rise," recent data from the Centers for Disease Control and Prevention show:

> **Fifteen percent of school-age boys have received an A.D.H.D. diagnosis, the data showed; the rate for girls was 7 percent. Diagnoses among those of high-school age – 14 to 17 – were particularly high, 10 percent for girls and 19 percent for boys. About one in 10 high-school boys currently takes A.D.H.D. medication, the data showed.**

Please note that the article is saying that about 19 percent of American high school boys have been diagnosed as having ADHD and that: **'About one in 10 high-school boys currently takes A.D.H.D. medication....'**

The fact that such a high proportion of boys have been targeted as a market for ADHD drugging over the past thirty years shows that the diagnosis has been illogical and illegitimate all along, since typical boyhood characteristics have obviously been used as justification for so much of the mass drugging.

Chapter Ten

Psychiatry's Diagnostic Manual and Their Insinuation into the Field of Medicine

The insinuation of the psychiatric profession into the field of medicine has been a long, gradual process that is still not totally complete. Some traditional medical doctors are skeptical and uncomfortable by their association with psychiatrists in the ranks of normal medicine. Many of them are dubious about or outright opposed to the damaging effects of standard psychiatric treatments to patients with brain operations, electric shock and drugs.

Until the latter part of the twentieth century, psychiatry was so differentiated from standard medicine that American health insurance companies would not pay for a lot of psychiatric treatments. However, in recent decades, this practice has changed and now many psychiatric treatments are covered by health insurance.

Psychiatry Has Taken On Some of the Characteristics of the Medical Profession

Psychiatry has taken on some of the characteristics of the medical profession. Psychiatrists attend medical schools and call themselves "doctors." They are part of the American Medical Association (AMA). The language they use to describe their activities portrays them as being in the field of medicine; they say they are "treating" "patients" for mental "illness."

American psychiatrists have created their *Diagnostic and Statistical Manual of Mental Disorders*. It looks like a medical manual of actual diseases, but, in fact, lists "mental disorders" that have never been actually located in patients' bodies. Instead, these "disorders" have simply been voted into the pages of the manual by committees of psychiatrists. The manual is primarily used to apply for insurance payments.

In a letter of December 4, 1998, addressed to the president of the American Psychiatric Association (APA), Loren R. Mosher, M.D., formally resigned from the organization. At one time Mosher had been very highly placed in the field of American psychiatry, in charge of the National Institute of Mental Health's Center for the Study of Schizophrenia. In this capacity, he conducted his own experiment throughout the 1970's known as the Soteria Project in which schizophrenic patients were treated with a minimal use of drugs, but good interpersonal relationships, and it was discovered that the project achieved higher cure rates, with less relapses back into schizophrenic states in later years, than the usual psychiatric treatments given to comparable schizophrenic patients, which relied heavily upon the use of psychiatric drugs. His findings were unpopular with some mainstream American psychiatrists and the manufacturers of the drugs that were being used in the conventional treatments of "mental patients."

In Loren Mosher's letter of resignation from the American Psychiatric Association was a paragraph discussing the *Diagnostic and Statistical Manual of Mental Disorders*, version number IV (commonly referred to as DSM-IV):

Finally, why must the APA pretend to know more than it does? DSM-IV is the fabrication upon which psychiatry seeks acceptance by medicine in general. Insiders know it is more of a political than scientific document. To its credit it says so – although its brief apologia is rarely noted. DSM-IV has become a bible and a money-making best seller – its major failings notwithstanding. It confines and defines practice, some take it seriously, others more realistically. It is the way to get paid. Diagnostic reliability is easy to attain for research projects. The issue is what do the categories tell us? Do they in fact accurately represent the person with a problem? They don't and can't, because there are no external validating criteria for

psychiatric diagnoses. There is neither a blood test nor specific anatomical lesions for any major psychiatric disorder. So where are we? APA as an organization has implicitly (sometimes explicitly as well) bought into a theoretical hoax. Is psychiatry a hoax – as practiced today? Unfortunately, the answer is mostly yes.

The Wide Gap Between Real Medicine and Psychiatry

Even though psychiatrists cloak themselves in similarities to the medical profession, there is a great deal of difference between the psychiatric profession and the profession of a real medical doctor.

A regular medical doctor is treating actual physical illness or disease. If a patient has a broken leg, then he obviously has something wrong with his body. It can be obvious to both the patient and the doctor, especially if x-rays are taken. A doctor can treat this specific physical illness by putting the bones of the patient's leg back together and wrapping it in a cast. If the doctor does his job correctly and the patient takes care of his leg, the leg heals in a few weeks and the illness in the patient's body is gone. The illness is "cured."

Similarly, if a person has strep throat due to a bacterial infection, a doctor can take a specimen from the patient's throat and under a microscope it can be seen that there are streptococcus bacteria in the specimen. The doctor can then treat the specific illness with an antibiotic, which will destroy the streptococcus bacteria and cure the patient's sore throat in a few days.

In both examples above we see that a medical doctor can actually locate the malfunction in the body of the person he is treating. The malfunction can be demonstrated to exist. Therein lies the difference between psychiatry and the field of standard, authentic medicine. In cases where a psychiatrist is treating a patient for a supposed "mental disorder," he cannot locate the "disorder" in the body of the patient he is treating.

If a person is labeled as "mentally ill" or as having a "mental disorder," the psychiatrist who is making the diagnosis is not doing it because of some specific abnormality that has been perceived in a person's body. He is making his diagnosis by simply looking at or just hearing about a person's behavior and deciding that it is odd, abnormal, politically incorrect or, as often happens in the case of a child diagnosed with ADHD, that it is unsuitable for a classroom. The fact that the so-called disorder cannot be actually located makes the diagnosis an arbitrary decision based on the opinion of the person doing the diagnosing.

Political Danger of Psychiatry's Arbitrary Diagnosing

Historically, the arbitrariness of psychiatric diagnoses being combined with the practice of involuntary commitment, which allows psychiatrists to forcibly incarcerate people in mental institutions or hospital wards against their will even when they have committed no crime, has opened the door to a great many instances of unfair, cruel incarcerations and psychiatric treatments. This combination of arbitrary diagnosing and involuntary commitment has also opened the door to the use of psychiatric diagnosis and treatment for political suppression. For instance, in Communist Russia, dissidents who spoke out against the oppression of their political system were routinely imprisoned in mental institutions and tortured with psychiatric drugs, sometimes for years. Some people will remember that in the late 1980's, one of Gorbachev's actions, when he came to power as General Secretary of the Communist Party in the Soviet Union, was to order that many people who had been forced into mental institutions in Russia for expressing political beliefs were to be released throughout the country.

Thus, it is obviously very dangerous to a society when psychiatric diagnoses can be used by governments as a basis for involuntary commitment, since they are based solely on arbitrary opinion, and the resulting treatments in the name of "health" can be used to destroy a person physically and mentally and can be used to crush his or her spirit.

Section III

Influences Behind the Drugging of Children for ADHD

Chapter Eleven

People Can Think ADHD Drugs Will Improve a Child's Academic Performance

Stimulants usually have similar effects on anybody, whether they have been labeled as having ADHD or not. When someone first takes methylphenidate or an amphetamine, they may experience an increase in energy, a greater ability to stay awake when they would usually be sleeping, greater ability to concentrate and they might feel more confident and even sort of invincible. However, after a few weeks or months of taking one of these drugs they would have to increase its dosages to maintain comparable levels of these characteristics. When a child is given an ADHD drug they often seem to improve in their academic performance initially, but the academic improvement is not long-term. The doctor who is prescribing the drug for a child labeled ADHD usually does not increase the dosages very much because he or she is aware of the drug's addictive qualities and some of the very dangerous adverse reactions that can occur with these substances.

Even the initial academic improvement that seems to occur with a child prescribed an ADHD stimulant is mainly improvement in concentration and more subdued classroom behavior, but is not necessarily improvement in understanding of material being studied. If a child who has been started on an ADHD drug doesn't know what the word "hypotenuse" means and is confused by a math problem using the word, he or she might be able to concentrate on the problem unwaveringly for 10 minutes, but it is likely they wouldn't be able to work out its answer correctly unless they were assisted in knowing the meaning of the word. ADHD drugs do not provide what is needed in situations like this. The child's ability to concentrate may be temporarily boosted at first, but not necessarily their comprehension.

Unfortunately, if children have been started on methylphenidate or an amphetamine drug, they can seem to be studiously concentrating and paying attention and appear to not require academic assistance. Thus, teachers and parents may not provide academic assistance to such children even when they need it, due to the child's studious appearance.

The full truth about the effects of stimulants on academic performance is often left out of promotional materials intended to get parents to use ADHD drugs on their children.

In an article titled "Ritalin Gone Wrong" in the January 28, 2012 *New York Times,* psychologist L. Alan Sroufe discussed the lack of benefit from ADHD drugs on academic performance even after a few weeks or months.

Attention-deficit drugs increase concentration in the short term, which is why they work so well for college students cramming for exams. But when given to children over long periods of time, they neither improve school achievement nor reduce behavior problems.

Toward the end of the same article, its author, L. Alan Sroufe, points out that studies show that ADHD drugs **'work for four to eight weeks....'**

The Phenomenon of Students Taking ADHD Drugs to Cram for Exams

ADHD drugs seem to heighten academic performance for students who ordinarily are not taking the drugs. For instance, there are high school and college students who take ADHD drugs in order to cram for exams, to be able to stay awake studying late into the night with increased concentration and to have the energy to take long exams the following day. The drugs do seem to give them an extra physical boost to study in this manner, although they don't necessarily help a student understand what they are studying better.

In the *New York Times* of June 9, 2012, there was an article titled "Risky Rise of the Good-Grade Pill" by Alan Schwarz. The article begins with a real example of a student pulling into his high school parking lot and "snorting" an ADHD drug to pep him up to take an exam:

The boy exhaled. Before opening the car door, he recalled recently, he twisted open a capsule of orange powder and arranged it in a neat line on the armrest. He leaned over, closed one nostril and snorted it.

Throughout the parking lot, he said, eight of his friends did the same thing.

Many of the students who jack their energy up using stimulants to get through exams are not ordinarily taking the stimulants on a regular basis day after day, as are the children who have been traditionally diagnosed ADHD. The students who use stimulants to cram for exams may not have a prescription, but are able to get the drugs from students who do have a prescription or they may be able to get the drugs by fooling a doctor into giving them a prescription. After the school exams are over, these students may go through a "crash" as they come down off the drugs and their bodies are recovering. It is also true that some of these students may become dependent on the drugs, thinking they need them to keep their grades up or to get into a college. They may find themselves taking higher and higher dosages as the months go by because their bodies' tolerances for the drugs continue to adjust and they can become more and more addicted. The more such students pull all-nighters, the more brain damage they are likely to be causing themselves. If they become addicted, they are likely to be shortening their own lives through lack of sleep, inadequate nutrition and an elevated heart rate, all being brought on at once.

The Double Standards for Athletes and Students

When our culture's professional, international and Olympic athletes take certain drugs we consider it cheating and illegal. Often the types of drugs they try to get away with are "performance enhancing" chemicals, like steroids. Sometimes, such as in the field of baseball, certain players have been known to take amphetamines, to give themselves extra energy and concentration for a game. Some have been known to do this on a regular basis.

Not only do we tend to look upon the drug-taking of our top athletes as cheating and illegal, we view them as setting very bad examples of behavior for our nation's youth.

However, when high school and college students take stimulants to cram and stay awake for exams, it has often been tolerated by many students and schools. Yet, it could be looked upon as a form of cheating as well. It is also often done illegally.

You would like to know, as a school administrator, that students could do their work on their own without resorting to illegal drug-taking to help them concentrate and stay up all night or several nights in a row. Likewise, as an employer, you would like to know that your employees can do their work on their own without amphetamines to prop them up physically and mentally. Perhaps it is important to you that your spouse or children are functioning as themselves, without a false, drug-induced facade that doesn't seem like the person you once knew.

Stimulant Drugs' Effects on Academic Performance for the Usual Student Labeled ADHD

Many people might think that millions of children are being labeled ADHD and prescribed stimulant drugs for long periods of time because the drugs will help the children understand more in school and lead to higher academic achievement. One will see ads for ADHD drugs in magazines that give the impression that children on ADHD drugs did better in school as a result of the drugs. Such a statement might have some truth to it, except that the advertiser leaves out the fact that the academic improvement is likely to be very short-lived, lasting only for a few weeks or months. Despite this reality, the parents or their insurance company or the taxpayers may be spending money on monthly prescriptions for a child's ADHD drugs for years, due to the false impression that the drugs are helping the child's academic performance during that time.

There have been many studies which showed that stimulant drugs failed to improve academic performance for those kids diagnosed and labeled as having ADHD and put on a stimulant medication on a daily basis for long periods of time.

When tests have been done about the effects of methylphenidate (Ritalin) and other psychiatric stimulants on the academic performance of children, one study after another showed that the drugs failed to improve academic performance over the long term. Some studies even indicated that these substances could worsen academic performance, especially when viewed over a long period. One of the studies given below mentions the drug "Diazepam," which is another name for the drug commonly known as Valium.

Some findings from a few of these studies undertaken in the 1970s and 1980s about the effects of stimulants on academic performance are presented here:

The belief that long-term drug intervention will continue to be of value or produce better outcome in hyperactive children has not been substantiated by this or other studies.

"A Four-Year Follow-up Study of the Effects of Methylphenidate on the Behavior and Academic Achievement of Hyperactive Children," Linda Charles and Richard Schain, *Journal of Abnormal Child Psychology,* December, 1981.

There have now been at least seven independent investigations of the stimulants in various groups of children with learning problems. Several types of reading assessments have been used as well as different

doses and varying periods of administration. However, none of these studies has been able to demonstrate consistent improvement in academic achievement … it seems reasonable to conclude for the present that stimulants have no clear role to play in specific learning difficulties.

"Methylphenidate and Diazepam in Severe Reading Retardation," Michael G. Aman, Ph.D. and John S. Werry, M.D., *Journal of the American Academy of Child Psychology*, 1982.

Ritalin and other Psychiatric Stimulants May Actually Worsen Academic Performance

There were studies indicating that administering Ritalin or other psychiatric stimulants to children could actually worsen their academic performance. Some of their findings and conclusions are given here:

Furthermore, the ideal dose for the suppression of conduct problems may actually impair cognitive performance (e.g., Swanson, Kinsbourne, Roberts, & Zucker 1978) or neutralize beneficial cognitive effects (Sprague & Sleater 1977) which, theoretically, could negate any beneficial effect on academic

achievement or even exacerbate the child's learning problems.

"Effects of Stimulant Drugs on Academic Performance in Hyperactive and Learning Disabled Children," by Kenneth D. Gadow, Ph.D., *Journal of Learning Disabilities,* May, 1983.

The present results suggest that continued use of Ritalin and possibly other drugs to control hyperactivity may result in compliant but academically incompetent students. Surely the goal of school is not to make children into docile robots either by behavior techniques or by medication.

The control of hyperactivity by medication, while effective, may be too costly to the child, in that it may retard his academic and social growth, a human cost that society and schools can ill afford.

"A Behavioral-Educational Alternative to Drug Control of Hyperactive Children," Ayllon, Layman and Kandel, *Journal of Applied Behavior Analysis,* Summer, 1975.

Teachers and Parents Often Believe Students on ADHD Drugs Are Doing Better Academically When Actually They Aren't

Another interesting thing about some of these early studies was that the researchers noticed that both teachers and parents would think that their students/children were doing better academically as a result of taking stimulants, yet when they were tested, the students would usually not be demonstrating increased academic performance. However, the teachers and parents would adopt this misconception because when the students were drugged they seemed to be more studious and attentive in their classrooms and homes.

A very important observation in these studies was that this misconception on the part of the teachers and parents could lead to the children being passed over for help that they really needed in their schoolwork. The following passages from studies done in the 1970s and 1980s highlight this point:

> **It is common for parents and teachers of methyphenidate-treated children to report marked improvement in school performance. Yet attempts to document these observations have not succeeded; and it is now generally believed that academic improvement is not associated with methylphenidate treatment.**

"Effects of Methylphenidate in Combination with Reading Remediation," Rachel Gittelman, Donald Klein and Ingrid Feingold, *Journal of Child Psychology and Psychiatry,* April, 1983.

Teachers and parents may mistakenly assume the behavioral improvements to be indicative of, or associated with, academic gains.

This explanation suggests the rather disturbing possibility that stimulant medications, while rendering hyperactive children more manageable and less disruptive, may lead teachers to overlook basic academic disabilities. The improvement in behavior may reduce the probability that these children will receive needed educational assistance in the classroom.

"Do Stimulant Drugs Improve the Academic Performance of Hyperkinetic Children," Russell A. Barkley and Charles E. Cunningham, *Clinical Pediatrics,* January, 1978

Effects of Ritalin upon scholastic achievement of 18 academically deficient

children were studied, in an attempt to validate findings of an earlier study of similar design. Results, in keeping with the previous research, indicate that while Ritalin affects behavior, it does not enhance learning, and may in fact mask academic problems.

"Effects of Ritalin on Underachieving Children," by Herbert and Ellen Rie, Stewart and Ambuel, *American Journal of Orthopsychiatry,* April, 1976.

To Summarize

Over the past forty years there have been numerous scientific studies undertaken to ascertain if Ritalin and other psychiatric stimulants improved academic performance in children. Often, the studies were conducted in the hopes that they would. However, one study after another failed to produce the desired outcome. As Gerald Coles stated in his book, published in 1987, *The Learning Mystique, A Critical Look at "Learning Disabilities"*:

Worst of all for drug advocates, whether the studies were short or long term, whether they met basic scientific criteria or not, all conclusions converged: "stimulant drugs have little, if any, impact on…long-term academic outcome."

It seems to be the case that children put on stimulant drugs who then appear to concentrate better and be more attentive in class, at least initially, and who are easier to manage in the classroom, are given higher grades and more glowing report cards by their teachers, even when their actual academic performance in terms of understanding and application has not been improved.

In spite of the temporary nature of academic improvement resulting from drugging children with stimulants, advertisements for ADHD drugs often speak in more general and deceptive terms about how the drugs improve academic performance. A great deal of money has been and is currently being wasted on ADHD drugs due to the delusion that the drugs are going to result in long-term academic benefit for the children.

The Placebo Factor in ADHD Drugging

There is another factor which must be occurring regarding the effects of ADHD drugs and that is the placebo effect, where one thinks they are doing better because they have swallowed a pill which they believe will make them somehow better. This phenomenon surely applies to some of the students given the drugs. But also, in a sense, both the teachers and parents of children given ADHD drugs may have a similar effect, in that they have also been led to believe the drugs are helping the children learn and understand, and because the children appear to be more studious and attentive once drugged, the grownups may also believe the children are doing better in their academic performance.

Negative Effects on Scholastic Performance Coincident with Use of ADHD Drugs

A more recent article about the effects of ADHD drugs on academic performance in children was published in the Journal *Nature* on February 12, 2014. The title of the article was "Medication: The smart-pill oversell," subtitled "Evidence is mounting that medication for ADHD doesn't make a lasting difference to schoolwork or achievement." It was written by Katherine Sharpe. In the article, it was noted that in a study in Quebec the use of the ADHD drug methylphenidate on students was coincident with higher rates of academic and behavior problems:

> **In 2013, a team of economists published a study examining the effects of a policy change in Quebec that resulted in thousands of children being given prescriptions for methylphenidate. The authors found that children who began taking it actually did worse at school and were more likely to drop out than those with similar levels of symptoms who did not receive drugs. Girls taking the drug had more emotional problems, and both sexes reported worse relationships with their parents.**

Obtaining Copies of Such Medical and Scientific Studies

Often, one can obtain summaries of such medical and scientific studies as those given in this chapter and elsewhere in this book by simply googling their titles. These summaries are referred to as "abstracts." To get the full articles that appeared in medical and scientific journals, one may be able to obtain them by going to a local medical university library.

Another way to obtain them is by going to a local library that is part of a network of libraries in one's area. Sometimes these library networks have one or more medical libraries in their network and by specifying which study you are requesting they can locate it and have it emailed to you.

The more people are aware of the studies the better.

As stated earlier, they are not always easy to read for one not familiar with their medical and scientific terminology. However, by using a dictionary they can still be understood by most readers. By looking over the studies relating to children's stunted body growth, probable brain damage and lack of academic improvement from children taking ADHD stimulant drugs, one can make up one's own mind as to the desirability of this widespread practice in our society.

Chapter Twelve

Diagnosing and Drugging Children for ADHD Is Profitable

We know there is evidence that stimulants generally don't improve academic performance in the long run for students labeled ADHD and put on the drugs for long periods of time at prescribed doses.

We know that the ADHD drugs can create numerous adverse effects upon the body, including stunted growth.

We know that it can be reasonably assumed that the use of psychiatric stimulants may adversely affect the hearts of users and possibly shorten the life span of many of the individuals they are administered to.

We know that there is evidence that stimulants may cause permanent brain damage, such as brain shrinkage and separation along the furrows on the surface of the brain, a process known as sulcal widening, and that they may cause neurological disabilities.

We know that ADHD drugs can cause a host of psychological side effects, including in some cases psychosis. Also, by the mere act of telling a child he has to take an ADHD drug, we may be causing him to conclude that there is something wrong with himself and that he can't succeed in life on his own.

We know that methylphenidate and amphetamines that are given to children for ADHD are rated as Schedule II drugs by the Drug Enforcement Administration because of their addictive qualities and likelihood of being abused.

We know that these drugs are indeed being abused on a large scale by students in schools and colleges throughout America while federal and state governments are spending millions of dollars to convince American children to "say no to drugs."

We know that the phrase "Attention Deficit Hyperactivity Disorder" was agreed upon by a committee of psychiatrists rather than being a real disease discovered in a person's body, and that the committee thought it should be included as one of the hundreds of mental disorders in the American Psychiatric Association's *Diagnostic and Statistical Manual of Mental Disorders,* which they use to apply for insurance payments.

We know that the diagnosing of ADHD is done by opinion, not physical, medical testing, and that it is often done within an initial visit with a psychiatrist or other prescriber.

We know that psychiatrists are already drugging a massive number of children labeled as having Attention Deficit Hyperactivity Disorder in the United States, Europe, Australia and some other countries, and that the vast majority of them are boys, and that the characteristics of being a boy are considered to be the symptoms of the presence of a mental disease by many people who are indoctrinated in ADHD presumptions.

We know that hundreds of thousands of diagnoses of ADHD have been occurring with the youngest children in classes, mainly because these children have behaved less maturely than the older children in the classes and because ADHD diagnoses are done by opinion rather than real, physical, medical testing.

So why are psychiatrists drugging children with psychiatric stimulants on a wholesale basis in America, Europe, Australia and other parts of the world?

The answer, at first glance, is simple: we are drugging certain children in our countries to make them less distracting and bothersome to others in their lives, especially in their classrooms and homes. In short, psychiatric stimulants are being used as sort of chemical straightjackets for kids. They don't actually keep them from moving their arms, but they may cause them to move around less, at least for a while after they are started on the drugs.

However, there are a lot of other contributing factors that are bringing about the wholesale drugging of children in our society. Primary among them is there is a lot of money to be made in the child-drugging industry.

Many mental health professionals and pharmaceutical companies stand to gain from the diagnosing and drugging of children for ADHD. A few of these professions are mentioned here.

Psychiatrists Can Make a Lot of Easy Money When They Label Children ADHD

When a child is brought to a typical psychiatrist to see if he has ADHD, it is almost a foregone conclusion that the child will be diagnosed as having the so-called mental disorder. There are no medical tests involved in the diagnosis. The psychiatrist can simply render an opinion that a child has ADHD and have a mother coming back for prescription refills month after month. A doctor can see dozens of clients like this each day and bill for every visit for a new prescription.

Unfortunately, many of these practitioners often give little attention to such children's home situations, schooling circumstances, nutritional deficiencies and personal lives. These are given little care and attention in favor of treating unsubstantiated "chemical imbalances" in the children's brains that are never found, measured or quantified.

The Pharmaceutical Companies Who Make ADHD Drugs Get Tremendous Amounts of Business from the Child-Drugging Market

Obviously, the drug companies producing ADHD drugs have reaped major profits. According to a *New York Times* article of Dec 14, 2013, by Alan Schwarz, titled "The Selling of Attention Deficit Disorder," **'Sales of stimulant medication in 2012 were nearly $9 billion, more than**

five times the $1.7 billion a decade before, according to the data company IMS Health.'

These drug companies do a lot of advertising of their ADHD drugs, such as with ads found in magazines targeted toward women readers, ads in publications read by doctors, ads on the internet, etc. They also do a lot of promoting to doctors at medical conventions and meetings. They spend a lot of money on seminars for doctors about how good and preferable their drugs are. They also spend a lot of money sending representatives from their companies to visit doctors to indoctrinate them about their drugs and give them gifts and expensive inducements.

Mental Health "Experts" Get Paid to Lecture Teachers, School Psychologists, Social Workers, Nurses and Others about ADHD

American teachers and other professionals in the mental health and medical fields are usually required to take continuing education courses after they have graduated from colleges with Bachelors, Masters and Doctorate degrees. They are often expected to attain a certain quota of credits in continuing education courses year after year as a requirement for keeping their professional certificates considered valid.

Many of the continuing education seminars that teachers are required to take contain information about psychological theories and approaches. These theories often come and go in waves of popularity. However, one subject which continues to be addressed by continuing education seminar leaders and "experts" year after year is ADHD, how to spot it in students, how to deal with these students, how to teach them and when to get them sent to a practitioner for diagnosing and drugging.

School Psychologists / School Adjustment Counselors and Social Workers Have Jobs Relating to Kids Being Labeled ADHD and Administered Drugs

School Psychologists, School Adjustment Counselors and mental health professionals of one kind or another are now posted directly in American schools all over the United States. Although the migration of these professions into U.S. schools had been going on gradually for several decades, it has now reached a point of being status quo in almost all public and many private schools throughout the country. These professionals often become participants in the effort to drug schoolchildren. While they may not actually prescribe the drugs the children are given, they are often involved in recommendations to parents and doctors that lead to children being drugged.

Such people are also often present when several school personnel meet with or gang up on a mother or a husband and wife to tell them that their child appears to have ADHD and should be taken to a doctor for evaluation and treatment. Of course, the treatment is very often drugging.

Chapter Thirteen

Drug Companies Reward Psychiatrists and Doctors Who Prescribe and Promote Their Drugs

This topic deserves a book itself. Many consumers of psychiatric and medical drugs don't realize that their doctors are getting paid financial benefits directly from drug companies when they prescribe the companies' drugs. It is very common these days for drug companies to send drug company representatives to visit doctors and drop off free gifts for them.

The drug companies procure the prescription records of doctors so they know how much each doctor is prescribing various drugs. The gifts from the drug companies to the doctors can range from pens and note pads to free tickets to sports games, free dinners at restaurants or paid trips to expensive resorts. They can also be in the form of monetary payments to doctors who will recommend a particular drug to other doctors or will give speeches promoting a drug at conventions or will agree to be a consultant to a drug company or will agree to have their name associated with a drug research study or will do a drug research study for a drug company. It is quite common for a doctor to receive tens of thousands of dollars a year from drug companies, completely in addition to the money he gets from fees he charges patients or pay he gets from a hospital. Some doctors receive hundreds of thousands of dollars a year from drug companies, especially if they agree to do research for them, become drug company consultants and/or give promotional speeches about drugs to large audiences of doctors.

Evidence of Psychiatrists Taking Highest Amounts of Drug Company Gifts

According to a *New York Times* article on July 12, 2008, titled "Psychiatric Group Faces Scrutiny Over Drug Industry Ties" by Benedict Carey and Gardiner Harris, there was evidence that the type of doctors who tend to average the highest amounts in payments from drug companies are psychiatrists:

> **While data on industry consulting arrangements are sparse, state officials in Vermont reported that in the 2007 fiscal year, drug makers gave more money to psychiatrists than to doctors in any other specialty. Eleven psychiatrists in the state received an average of $56,944 each. Data from Minnesota, among the few other states to collect such information, show a similar trend.**

In an article titled "Dollars for Docs Mints a Millionaire," by Tracy Weber and Charles Ornstein, on March 11, 2013 on the ProPublica website, it was noted that among all of the specialists in medicine getting paid by drug companies **'half of the top earners are from a single specialty: psychiatry.'**

In the November 24, 2011 *New York Times* was an article titled "Payments to Doctors by Pharmaceutical Companies Raise Issues of Conflicts" by reporters Emily Ramshaw and Ryan Murphy. It gives one an idea of the magnitude of the financial inducements drug companies lavish upon doctors to encourage them to prescribe their drugs. For example, the article stated:

> **From 2009 to early 2011, at least 25,000 Texas physicians and researchers received a combined $57 million - and probably far more - in cash payments, research money, free meals, travel and other perks, according to data culled from 12 drug companies and provided by the nonprofit investigative news organization ProPublica.**

U.S. Senator Exposes Boston Psychiatrists Receiving Millions in Drug Company Payments

Some of the most glaring examples of psychiatrists taking payments from drug companies were found in Boston. In 2008, U.S. Senator Charles E. Grassley was investigating the phenomenon of consulting fees being paid to doctors by drug companies. There were two psychiatrists at a major hospital in Boston who he found had each been paid 1.6 million dollars over several years from drug companies and another psychiatrist from the same hospital who had been paid one million. A *New York Times* article on June 8, 2008, by Gardiner Harris and Benedict Carey titled "Researchers Fail to Report Full Drug Pay" gave the following information concerning one of these psychiatrists named Joseph Biederman:

A world-renowned Harvard child psychiatrist whose work has helped fuel an explosion in the use of powerful antipsychotic medicines in children earned at least $1.6 million in consulting fees from drug makers from 2000 to 2007 but for years did not report much of this income to university officials, according to information given Congressional investigators.

An associate of Biederman, Dr. Timothy Wilens, also received $1.6 million from drug companies during the same time period. Another of his associates, Dr. Thomas Spencer, received $1 million from drug companies during the same period.

Dr. Biederman has been one of the leading psychiatrists in the United States at assisting drug companies who make ADHD drugs to advertize and sell their products. According to a December 14, 2013 *New York Times* article titled "The Selling of Attention

Deficit Disorder," by Alan Schwarz: **'Findings from Dr. Biederman's dozens of studies on the disorder and specific brands of stimulants have filled the posters and pamphlets of pharmaceutical companies that financed the work.'**

Dr. Biederman has recently been coming under fire for researching the use of very strong drugs known as antipsychotics on young children, and his "findings" and pronouncements about the drugs have had a strong influence on the increased use of antipsychotics on children across America.

The drugs known as antipsychotics have been found to substantially shorten the lives of mental patients and elderly, and we can assume that they would be very harmful to the health of children. One of the ways the antipsychotics bring patients to an early demise is that they often cause rapid weight gain, followed by diabetes. They cause many other side effects as well.

Antipsychotics Even Used to Treat Children Labeled ADHD

Antipsychotics are very strong drugs. Traditionally they have been used to control patients in mental hospitals. Examples of older antipsychotics are drugs like Thorazine and Haldol, both of which are still in common use today. In recent years, a whole new batch of antipsychotics have been introduced to the market. The reason they are being briefly mentioned in this work is the fact that some of these very strong toxins are now being given to children, sometimes at very young ages, as treatment for supposed ADHD.

On August 9, 2012, an article titled "Antipsychotics Prescribed to Treat ADHD In More Children And Teens, New Study Finds" by Cathleen Pearson appeared in the *Huffington Post*. The article stated:

> **The number of children and teens taking antipsychotic medications has skyrocketed in recent years, with psychiatrists prescribing the drugs in nearly one-in-three visits with youth, a new study found.**
>
> **The drugs are not only being prescribed for schizophrenia and bipolar disorder, but also for the commonly diagnosed attention deficit hyperactivity disorder (ADHD).**

On March 17, 2014, Express Scripts Lab released their findings from a study of "pharmacy claims of more than 400,000 individuals...." The title of the article is "Turning Attention to ADHD: U.S. Medication Trends for Attention Deficit Hyperactivity Disorder." The article was written David Muzina, M.D. Among the many findings of this study was the following: '**The prescribing of antipsychotic treatments is exceptionally high among those treated for ADHD (12% vs. 4% of non-ADHD medication users)....**'

A few data about antipsychotic drugs are given below, not only because they are now being prescribed for some children with ADHD, but also because they are known to gradually kill patients and the promotion of their expanded use on children was apparently largely brought about through sizable drug company payments to several psychiatrists.

Antipsychotic Drugs Shorten the Lives of Elderly

To give an idea of how toxic antipsychotic drugs are and how inappropriate they could be for children, the following data are presented.

In April, 2005, the FDA ordered black box warnings on antipsychotics. In an article written by Gardiner Harris titled "Popular Drugs for Dementia Tied to Deaths" in the April 12, 2005 *New York Times,* the reason for the FDA's announcement was explained.

The Food and Drug Administration said that it had analyzed the results of 17 placebo-controlled trials involving the drugs, which are known as atypical antipsychotics. The agency found that elderly patients with dementia who were given the pills were 1.6 to 1.7 times as likely to die as those given placebos.

The point is, these drugs have been found to hasten the deaths of patients. Should these toxins be forced on children, including very young children?

Antipsychotics and the Extraordinary, Early Deaths of Mental Patients

The fact that mental patients tend to die prematurely in America is nothing new to some people who work in the mental health field dealing directly with patients. It is something that they have been observing for decades and sometimes comment upon.

The following is another piece of information that bears out this point of antipsychotics shortening the life span of patients. In October 2006, the findings from a very large study about the treatment of mental patients in America was released. It was titled "Morbidity and Mortality in People with Serious Mental Illness." The study was conducted for the National Association of State Mental Health Program Directors. For the report, the treatment of mental patients was researched in eight different states of the U.S.A. On page 11 of the report, in a section titled **'Overview - The Problem,'** it was stated:

People with serious mental illness served by our public mental health systems die, on average, 25 years earlier than the general population.

Please note that the finding said **'25 years earlier.'** (The researchers were using 76 years as the average age of death by the general population and they found the mental patients dying, on average, at age 51.)

One of the main reasons for these early deaths is given on page 6 of the study:

> ...the second generation antipsychotic medications have become more highly associated with weight gain, diabetes, dyslipidemia, insulin resistance and the metabolic syndrome....

In summary, antipsychotic drugs appear to be life-shortening to very significant degrees and it is astounding that children are now being made to take these toxins, especially when their bodies and brains are in the process of developing.

Antipsychotics Found to Accelerate Loss of Brain Tissue in Patients

A famous researcher, Dr. Nancy Andreasen, spent years analyzing the brains of patients labeled "schizophrenic" using brain scans. In an interview published in *The New York Times* of September 16, 2008, titled "A Conversation with Nancy C. Andreasen" by Claudia Dreifus, Andreasen said, **'Another thing we've discovered is that the more drugs you've been given, the more brain tissue you lose.'** She found that some of the patients being treated for schizophrenia were losing brain tissue at a rate of about one percent a year, faster than the general population at the same ages. The one percent seems small, but over time becomes very significant; for example, over a period of 20 years a patient could lose 20

116

percent of his or her brain, especially if they were taking antipsychotics during this time.

In the "Results" from a study authored by Nancy Andreasen and 4 other researchers, published in the February, 7, 2011 issue of *Archives of General Psychiatry*, titled "Long-term Antipsychotic Treatment and Brain Volumes: A Longitudinal Study of First-Episode Schizophrenia," were the following statements:

Greater intensity of antipsychotic treatment was associated with indicators of generalized and specific brain tissue reduction after controlling for effects of three other predictors. More antipsychotic treatment was associated with smaller gray matter volumes. Progressive decrement in white matter volume was most evident among patients who received more antipsychotic treatment.

This was a major study done over many years. The finding that the antipsychotics cause loss of brain tissue is another reason they should not be given to children whose brains are growing and developing. You don't want children having their brains failing to grow properly because of a drug or multiple drugs they are taking.

For all the above reasons—the fact that the antipsychotics have been shown to hasten the deaths of elderly patients, that they are a major factor in bringing about the very early deaths of mental patients, and finally that they are associated with significant loss of brain tissue—the drugs known as antipsychotics should not be being given to children, or probably any human being.

Unfortunately, statistics are showing there has been a tremendous growth in the use of antipsychotics for children in recent years, even for children labeled ADHD.

Psychiatrists' Prescribing Habits Influenced

It appears that some drug companies have found gifting and payments to psychiatrists to be very successful in causing increased prescriptions and drug sales, even of very strong, toxic, psychiatric drugs for small children.

In the *New York Times* article of July 12, 2008, "Psychiatric Group Faces Scrutiny Over Drug Industry Ties," by Benedict Carey and Gardiner Harris, the authors noted a correlation between the amount of money being paid by drug companies to psychiatrists and the amount of antipsychotics they were prescribing for children:

An analysis of Minnesota data by The New York Times last year found that on average, psychiatrists who received at least $5,000 from makers of newer-generation antipsychotic drugs appear to have written three times as many prescriptions to children for the drugs as psychiatrists who received less money or none.

118

Thus, one can see that it is likely that many psychiatrists who are prescribing ADHD drugs or other drugs to children might not be doing so because they think it is best for their patients, but rather because it is best for their personal incomes.

When doctors are asked about the influence of gifts and money from drug companies on their prescribing habits, it is common for them to respond that the gifts and payments do not influence their treatment decisions about patients. However, studies have shown this to be untrue, at least in many cases. Some good examples of this phenomenon of doctors denying being influenced by drug company gifts and yet markedly changing their prescribing patterns after the receipt of the gifts can be seen in an article titled "Prescribing Under the Influence," by E. Haavi Morreim.

Obviously, drug companies have found the practice of giving hundreds of millions of dollars in gifts and money to doctors across the country to be successful in driving up sales of their drugs. Otherwise, they wouldn't be doing it. They know they can get the money back from insurance companies, Medicaid and Medicare.

Shedding Some Light on Drug Company Payments to Doctors

In March 2010 a piece of federal legislation for the United States was passed into law known as The Sunshine Act, since it will shed some light on the financial rewards and inducements drug companies and medical device makers give to psychiatrists and other doctors to influence which treatments they apply to their patients.

As a result of this piece of legislation, drug companies are now mandated by the U.S. Government to keep exact records of the gifts they give to doctors, whether the gifts are small or large. Starting in September 2014, there are supposed to be reports available to the broad public concerning which doctors were receiving gifts from drug companies and medical device makers, the value of the gifts and what sort of gifts they were. The program is known as the National Physician Payment Transparency Program.

To give credit where it is due, Senator Chuck Grassley co-authored this piece of legislation with another Senator, Herb Kohl.

With the new law, gifts and payments to psychiatrists and doctors from drug companies will still occur, but the practice may be somewhat restrained due to a light of truth piercing the shadows surrounding this development in American medicine.

Chapter Fourteen

U.S. Government Program Rewards Parents for Drugging their Children

There is a United States government program known as Supplemental Security Income (SSI) that was originally designed to provide financial assistance to elderly, blind and disabled people in financial need. Today, it is mostly used to pay monthly checks to poor parents whose children have been diagnosed with a "mental disorder" such as ADHD. The checks can be quite substantial, for as much or more than $700.00 per month per child. For instance, if a single mother can get 3 of her children labeled with ADHD or some other mental disorder label and then put on psychiatric drugs, she can make approximately $2100.00 each month from the taxpayers without having to do much more than fill out the initial paperwork and see a doctor once a month to get prescription refills. The free SSI payments from the government can be spent on food, housing and clothing. This can free up a parent's finances to use their other sources of income to buy televisions, jewelry, make car payments or whatever the parent wants. Taking a prescribed medication has almost become a prerequisite for such children to qualify for the payments. Consequently, hundreds of thousands of children are being drugged with psychiatric drugs daily in the U.S., largely due to the financial inducements of this government program.

When a family is approved to receive Supplemental Security Income for a child, the child is usually approved to have his or her medical costs covered by Medicaid. Thus, the costs of the parents' visits to doctors each month to get prescription refills and the costs of the monthly supplies of drugs for their kids are automatically covered by Medicaid, which means these expenses each month for each family doing this all around the U.S. are also being covered by the taxpayers.

Thus, for the families who qualify for Supplemental Security Income, the taxpayers are covering the costs of the monthly SSI checks for the patients, the costs of all the monthly doctor visits to get prescriptions renewed for the children's drugs and the costs of the drugs themselves to be purchased at pharmacies.

Supplemental Security Income Gets Some Exposure Due to the Death of 4-Year-Old Rebecca Riley

The Supplemental Security Income program was brought to public attention when a four-year-old girl named Rebecca Riley died on December 13, 2006, due to being overdosed on psychiatric drugs by her parents.

She had been labeled ADHD and bipolar by a Dr. Kayoko Kifuji, a psychiatrist in Boston. Rebecca had been put on psychiatric drugs from the age of two.

Her two older siblings had already been given mental disorder labels and were already being drugged. The parents were obtaining SSI payments for these two oldest children. They were in the process of trying to get an additional, monthly SSI payment for their 4 year-old daughter when they overdosed her.

According to *The Boston Globe* website Boston.com on January 25, 2010, in an article by Patricia Wen titled "Psychiatrist admits she approved higher drug dosage in Riley trial," during the trial, the following occurred:

While being questioned by the prosecutor, Dr. Kayoko Kifuji acknowledged that when she first met Rebecca Riley, at age 2, she had initially diagnosed her with having attention-deficit hyperactivity disorder after only a one-hour meeting. She authorized the mother to give one prescription tablet of clonidine, a sedative, each night.

Later Dr. Kifuji decided the little girl was bipolar and prescribed more drugs for her including an antipsychotic drug.

Another interesting point that relates to information from the previous chapter is one of Dr. Kifuji's early justifications for prescribing strong psychiatric drugs for this very young child. It was stated in a Boston.com article of June 17, 2007, titled "Backlash on bipolar diagnoses in children," by Scott Allen:

Still, many wondered why a girl so young was being treated in the first place with Clonidine and two other psychiatric drugs, including one not approved for children's use. Riley's psychiatrist has said she was influenced by the work of Biederman and his protege, Dr. Janet Wozniac.

The death of 4-year-old Rebecca Riley struck a chord with many people because it was so outrageous to find a two-year-old put on a strong psychiatric drug for ADHD, and later, additional strong drugs apparently for the purpose of acquiring more SSI payments from the taxpayers.

The poisoning death of Rebecca Riley by psychiatric drugs caused other psychiatrists and doctors to become upset with Dr. Biederman, since he had been a foremost proponent for the use of antipsychotic drugs on very young children. A statement by one of these doctors named Lawrence Diller was published in the *Boston Globe* on June 19, 2007, titled "Misguided standards of care." A paragraph from the article is given here:

Naming names in medicine is just not done very often - and I knew the personal and professional risks I was taking. Yet I felt compelled to name Joseph Biederman, head of the Massachusetts General Hospital's

Pediatric Psychopharmacology clinic, as morally culpable in providing the "science" that allowed Rebecca to die.

According to a news story titled "Father Seeks New Trial in Daughter's 2006 Overdose Death," on November 29, 2013, by Associated Press Legal Affairs Writer Denise Lavoie, prosecutors in the legal case against Rebecca Riley's parents stated that the parents had fabricated her mental disorder symptoms for the purpose of acquiring additional benefits on their third child.

More Exposure of SSI

A three-part series was published in *The Boston Globe* from December 12-14, 2010, concerning the effects of SSI checks to supplement the income of families with children labeled with mental disorders. The title of the series was "A legacy of unintended side effects." The author of the three-part series was *Boston Globe* award-winning reporter Patricia Wen. A lot of research was done for this illuminating series of articles, including interviews with many parents and children of families receiving SSI checks. This passage from the first of the three articles in the series gives an overview of some of the findings of the research for the articles:

And once a family gets on SSI, it can be very hard to let go. The attraction of up to $700 a month in payments, and the near-automatic Medicaid coverage that comes with

SSI approval, leads some families to count on a child's remaining classified as disabled, even as his or her condition may be improving. It also leads many teenage beneficiaries to avoid steps - like taking a job - that might jeopardize the disability check.

Amazingly, there seems to be no genuine, good reason why a parent should be paid approximately $700.00 a month from the taxpayers just for having a child who has been labeled as having ADHD. And the amount of the monthly payments continually goes up as the years go by. Of course, the payments encourage the practice, so that more and more children will be put on drugs and their parents will not want to take actions to stop this, as they become accustomed to a lifestyle with free money from the taxpayers.

It is important to realize the role that the ADHD diagnosis and other psychiatric diagnoses play in the country's rapidly expanding SSI program. If you have a government program that pays people large sums of money for getting their children diagnosed with a supposed mental disorder like ADHD and the "diagnosis" can be done simply on the basis of a parent making a few comments to a psychiatrist about their child's behavior, you are going to be getting a lot of fraud and the taxpayers are once again going to be taken to the cleaners, as the saying goes.

Then there are the physical and psychological costs to the child and the moral costs to those involved for being dishonest and committing harm. However, this is often what the government program rewards in many Supplemental Security Income cases, particularly some of those based on "mental disorders," such as ADHD.

Chapter Fifteen

Schools Have Been Turned into a Main Marketing Tool for the Psychiatric Child-Drugging Industry

The Psychiatric Medicalization of American Education

A positioning that psychiatry constantly works to cultivate in the minds of American citizens and politicians is that they are part of the field of medicine. This position in the public mind enables them to carry some of the prestige of a regular doctor, to collect health insurance payments, to benefit from government disbursements for public health programs and to prescribe drugs.

The field of psychiatry doesn't position naturally into the field of medicine. It is an awkward association based mainly on assumptions and opinions, but little scientific evidence. It is doubtful if one could find another mainstream academic subject so filled with false information, pet theories, conflicting opinions, lack of workable technology and so devoid of axioms as one would expect to find in any field of real science.

The awkward association of psychiatry and the field of actual medicine has caused other awkward distortions in the field of education. In 1975, Congress passed the Education for All Handicapped Children Act, the purpose of which was to provide equal education to handicapped children, such as those who were blind, deaf and afflicted with real, physical diseases. Tacked on to the end of the definition of "handicapped children" in the bill was the additional category "children with specific learning disabilities," even though these supposed "disabilities" were generally not able to be located in the bodies of students. Nevertheless, this phrasing opened the door for psychiatrists and psychologists to get into the field of education and directly into schools to treat children.

Up to that time, the few medical professionals who worked in schools, such as school nurses, came to check on the students' physical bodies and left the educating to the teachers. But this new sort of medicine, psychiatry, became deeply involved in the processes of learning within the classrooms.

Since the passage of the Education for All Handicapped Children Act of 1975, the percentages of children with actual physical illnesses have stayed roughly the same. However, the percentages of children found to have "learning disabilities" has ballooned into a multi-billion dollar a year market for psychiatrists, psychologists, companies doing testing for "learning disabilities," disability experts, special education specialists, as well as regular doctors, pharmacists and pharmaceutical manufacturers. Numerous federal bills have since further consolidated the role of "mental health" in American schools.

Thus, today, we have the weird phenomenon of the medicalization of American education, another unnatural displacement of one body of ideas into another. What makes the whole phenomenon more unnatural is that the supposed "medicine," psychiatry, can't really prove that it is medicine because psychiatrists and psychologists can't find what they are supposedly treating in their patients' bodies, nor point to any physical cures in their patients' bodies once they have performed their treatments.

Consequently, mental health practitioners have had to do a lot of marketing and public relations in magazines, radio, television, newsprint and lobbying in the halls of power to convince the public that they are in the field of medicine and that their services should be used. Thus, one might see strange ads or billboards comparing ADHD to diabetes or similar assertions, trying to make the public think that a behavior is the same as a disease. A kid not paying attention in a class is not a disease.

One of American Psychiatry's Biggest Marketing Tricks

There is a part of the marketing of psychiatric and psychological services in America which is one of the biggest of all of them, and yet seems to go largely unnoticed—and that is that many of America's teachers have been made into a nationwide referral system for the psychiatric child-drugging market. This comment is not meant as an attack upon teachers, who often have very difficult jobs that are very important to the well-being of our society. This perversion of the role of teachers has been accomplished under the guise and cloak of health and medicine coming to the aid of the unfortunate "disabled" children in our society. But under the cloak, of course, is the psychiatrist with his bottles of amphetamines, antidepressants and life-shortening antipsychotic drugs.

American teachers are required to study psychology courses in order to graduate their teacher training. They are also required to take continuing education courses and seminars year after year, many of which have been about so-called "mental disorders" and mental "disabilities" they should expect to see in their students, including the supposed "symptoms" to watch for in their classrooms. Thus, when the supposed "symptoms" are displayed in a student, the child's teacher can report that he seems to have a "mental disorder" or "disability" and route him into the hands of someone who specializes in "mental health." In America today, there are psychologists posted within many schools and parents are often told by school personnel that their child should see a psychiatrist or doctor to see if he or she has ADHD or a "learning disability." It's very likely that the child will be put on one or more drugs if he or she is sent to a psychiatrist.

Creating this referral network out of America's teachers has created a gold mine for the mental health and pharmaceutical industries in America, producing literally millions upon millions of customers and billions upon billions of dollars of business and drug sales, making a flagrant exploitation of the educational system to go after a target market, the nation's children.

The school psychologists can be used to give children psychological testing and treatment and aid in the process of recommending to parents that their children be sent to a psychiatrist or regular doctor to be checked to see if they have ADHD or some other supposed mental disorder.

Consequently, today, millions of American children are taking psychiatric drugs daily. Many classrooms in the U.S. can have approximately 15% or more of their students on these sorts of drugs including ADHD amphetamine-type drugs, antidepressants, antipsychotics, tranquilizers, anti-anxiety drugs and various combinations of these. This constitutes a gigantic market for the mental health and pharmaceutical industries.

These children and their classmates are being taught that the solution to life's problems is drugs. Many of these children, now labeled with mental disorders, are destined to become life-long mental health clients.

Mental Health Screening — Casting Nets for Children to be Put on Drugs in Our Nation's Classrooms

One of the more sinister devices psychiatrists have devised is the practice known as mental health screening. A class of students may be given a survey to fill out. The survey will ask about the students' personal lives, their relations with others, their moods and attitudes. Once the surveys are done, many of the students will be interviewed for more information and many of these can become candidates for psychiatric diagnosing and drugging. This screening has actually been going on in the United States in many schools throughout the country. The practice has some similarity to a fishing trawler hauling a wide net in its wake seeking to catch a batch of fish to bring to market. The students being surveyed with mental health screening are not just prospects for ADHD drugging; they are prospects for drugging for depression, Post Traumatic Stress Disorder (PTSD), anxiety, worry, nervousness, lack of confidence, etc.

The Increasing Mental Health Labeling of School Children

Oddly enough, the American federal and state governments often display a marked tendency to reward non-production or disability in their citizenry. Perhaps this tendency is born out of compassion for those whose lives are difficult, but nevertheless the rewards tend to bring about greater numbers of the non-productive and seemingly disabled citizens. The most obvious place we have seen this tendency is in our welfare system. As shown in the previous chapter, we see it in the SSI (Supplementary Security Income) program which pays parents substantial monthly sums for getting their children labeled with mental disorders and drugged and we see the reluctance of the families to end off using the program when their children seem to no longer warrant the ADHD diagnosis.

In the field of American education, this tendency to reward non-productivity and disability (and to increase the prevalence of both) has been very pronounced. For instance, on a broad scale, one can note that the American SAT and other test scores declined for decades while federal monies and programs going to American education constantly expanded during the same time period. Both the national Verbal and Math SAT scores began trending downward coincident with the passage of the famous bill known as the Elementary and Secondary Education Act in 1965.

Another area where there has been gigantic growth due to federal monetary inducements has been in the field of "special education" for those diagnosed and labeled with some kind of "learning disability," such as Attention-Deficit Hyperactivity Disorder.

As stated above, in 1975, Congress passed the Education for All Handicapped Children Act. The idea behind the bill was to provide equal education to handicapped children, but included in the definition of "handicapped children" was the category of "children with specific learning disabilities." This phrasing opened the financial floodgates for psychiatry. It has also opened the doors for psychiatrists to step into the American educational picture with their growing lists of "learning disabilities" and "disorders," and their long lists of pills they claim help these supposed maladies. Though these "disabilities" and "mental disorders" have never been actually located in the bodies of children, they have been voted into the pages of the insurance manual of the American Psychiatric Association, *The Diagnostic and Statistical Manual of Mental Disorders*, enabling psychiatrists to collect Medicaid and private insurance payments for the writing of prescriptions for millions of children labeled with ADHD and other supposed mental disorders.

As could be expected, since the passage of the bill, the United States has not suffered a vast increase in the percentages of blind, deaf, and physically impaired children, but since there is no way to physically and scientifically verify if a child has ADHD or any "mental disorder," there was a virtual explosion of the numbers of children found to have "learning disabilities" and "disorders," even with a decrease in the number of students in public schools from the "baby boomer" days of the sixties and seventies. According to the April 24, 1984 edition of *Education Week*, the "learning disability" industry took off with a bang once the bill was passed:

Since the enactment in 1975 of the federal law guaranteeing handicapped

children the right to an education, the number of learning-disabled students receiving special services in the nation's schools has risen by 948,658 children to 1.7 million, a 119-percent increase over a seven year period. During that same time, overall enrollment in public schools dropped by about 11.5% according to federal statistics.

In their December 13, 1993 issue, *U.S. News and World Report* reported on the expansion of government-sponsored education programs since the passage of the federal bill known as the Individuals with Disabilities Education Act (IDEA):

Since the implementation of IDEA legislation, the number of students in special education has increased every year without exception. Today, there are 5 million special education students in the nation's schools—10 percent of all students enrolled.... Nationally, the bill for all special education services has rocketed from roughly $1 billion in 1977 to more than $30 billion today.

According to a Centers for Disease Control and Prevention (CDC) report from 2005, ADHD and Learning Disability (LD) diagnoses were still on the rise:

In 2003, approximately 16% of boys and 8% of girls aged 5-17 years had ever been diagnosed of ADHD or LD, according to

parental reports. Boys were three times more likely to have diagnoses of ADHD without LD. Boys were also more likely than girls to have LD diagnosed, either with or without ADHD.

A Centers for Disease Control and Prevention report from August 2011, listing key findings from a "National Health Interview Survey, 1998-2009", gave figures of the percentages of U.S. children labeled with ADHD diagnoses, but not combined with Learning Disability figures. Listed as a key finding was the following:

For the 2007-2009 period, an annual average of 9.0% of children aged 5-17 years had ever been diagnosed with ADHD—an increase from 6.9% in 1998-2000.

From 1998-2009, ADHD prevalence was higher among boys than girls: For boys, ADHD prevalence increased from 9.9% in 1998-2000 to 12.3% in 2007-2009, and for girls, from 3.6% to 5.5% during the same period.

It is also interesting to note that in both of the CDC reports above, boys were still approximately two and a half times as likely to be labeled ADHD as girls. This is a closer ratio than used to be the case which was about 9 boys to each girl. Nevertheless, these figures show that normal boy characteristics are still being used to label boys with mental disorders, as though the boy characteristics are symptoms of a disease. This should make the diagnosis laughable, except it is so tragic.

Also, the facts that in recent years over 12% of American boys between the age of 5 and 17 and millions of girls have been diagnosed with ADHD are staggering figures, when one considers that the majority of them have probably been drugged with dangerous and addictive drugs with numerous, serious side effects.

The *New York Times* reported on April 9, 2013, in an article by The Editorial Board, titled "Worry Over Attention Deficit Cases," about ADHD diagnoses specifically of American high school children:

Health providers diagnosed the disorder in 19 percent of high school boys and 10 percent of high school girls; about one in 10 high school boys currently takes prescription stimulants like Ritalin or Adderall to treat the disorder.

If one in ten of all high school boys in the United States are taking an ADHD stimulant drug on a daily basis, as well as millions of high school girls, one can see that this is a gigantic drug market that has been created. The above figures give a sense of the amount of business that using our nation's school systems has created for psychiatry's child-drugging market. They also show that this child-drug market is gradually being increased year after year.

Additionally, it should be realized that the ADHD drugs were gateway drugs that opened the doors to all manner of other drugging of children for depression, PTSD, Asperger's, bipolar, etc. They also opened the door for antipsychotics to be given to children, including very young ones, even though these drugs have been shown to shorten lives and markedly decrease brain tissue. Our nation's children are being exploited as a huge, psychiatric drug market and this is being largely accomplished through our schools.

Chapter Sixteen

Parents Can Be Threatened with Having Their Children Taken Away If They *Don't* Drug Them

In American society, there is another contributing influence to the wholesale drugging of schoolchildren that must be mentioned. It is actually quite common. Though some parents will never have heard of it, many other parents have, particularly those from poorer neighborhoods. It is the threat or actual use of seizure of a family's child or children by a state's Child Protective Services Agency. The Child Protective Services system is a national system, and each state has its own name for the agency in its particular state.

If a parent of a schoolchild is refusing to cooperate with school officials about drugging his or her child for ADHD, a school psychologist, social worker or even a teacher might accuse the parent of "medical neglect" and threaten the parent with having the child seized by agents from Child Protective Services. This is a threat of force to coerce the parent to cooperate. Sometimes the person threatening the parent may threaten to not only remove the child in question, but any of their other children as well. These are not always idle threats since it sometimes does happen. Such threats can be very unnerving to a parent.

There is an aspect about mental health that is a human rights issue and that is the fact that it is lawful in America for people to be seized and forcibly placed in a mental ward, and forcibly drugged without the consent of the victim, otherwise known as the "patient." This can occur even when the victim has not committed a crime or even a minor illegal act. The practice is known legally as "involuntary commitment." It can be done suddenly in a hospital or by police before there is any trial, use of a jury or hearing before a judge. An individual is seized, often with the help of hospital security guards, and forced into an institution or hospital ward. If the victim tries to escape or fights back or simply refuses to cooperate, multiple male individuals might force the individual to lie face down on the floor, hold him or her down and pull down their pants or garments while a nurse rams a hypodermic needle into one of their buttocks. The contents of the needle will be such a strong sedative that the victim will be rendered partially or more likely wholly unconscious in a few moments and he or she can then be easily rolled on a gurney into a locked seclusion room in a mental ward where they will wake up many hours later. After the forced incarceration and drugging, a "justice" action may occur in which a judge's consent for incarceration and treatment is obtained. It is also true

143

that sometimes consent from a judge is obtained before an involuntary commitment is committed.

This involuntary aspect or characteristic of mental health treatment seems to flavor other activities connected with it. One may experience a sense of coercion in the field of regular medicine sometimes from certain individual doctors or nurses. Since Child Protective Services is staffed with many individuals trained in mental health ideology and practices, it certainly has this coercive flavor. A parent may be at home with their child or children when suddenly people from Child Protective Services and police come to their home and forcibly seize a child or all of the children. The children are quickly brought to a Child Protective Services institution and very soon thereafter they may be diagnosed with one or more mental disorders and put on psychiatric drugs. The diagnosing of these kids happens soon after they have been forcefully seized and taken away from their parents, home, school, and friends, so they may be in an upset, anxious state when they are brought before the psychiatrist who does the diagnosing. It is appalling the amount of strong psychiatric drugs that are often forced on children in Child Protective Services. Though their home life may have been far from optimum, the treatment they might receive while in Child Protective Services custody can be even more abusive, particularly when they are drugged for years at a time with life-shortening, brain-shrinking antipsychotics combined with other toxic mixtures. The drugs and treatment they receive may physically and mentally ruin them.

The point is that the threat of Child Protective Services taking a parent's children away is a very coercive means to get parents to drug their children and it has been used for decades in some American public schools. It has often been used to force parents to drug their children for ADHD. Sometimes a social worker or person threatening the parents may accuse them of "medical neglect" for not putting their child on a drug for ADHD, despite the fact that there is no proof the child has any illness and despite the fact that once the child is put on a psychiatric drug, real physical damage and disease are likely to be caused to the child's body.

A sad case in point can be found at the website ritalindeath.com, as told by the father of a boy named Matthew:

> **Matthew's story started in a small town within Berkley, Michigan. While in first grade Matthew was evaluated by the school, who believed he had ADHD. The school social worker kept calling us in for meetings. One morning at one of those meetings while waiting for the others to arrive, Monica told us that if we refused to take Matthew to the doctor and get him on Ritalin, child protective services could charge us for neglecting his educational and emotional needs. My wife and I were intimidated and scared. We believed that there was a very real possibility of losing our children if we did not comply with the schools threats.**

Monica further explained ADHD to us, stating that it was a real brain disorder. She also went on to tell us that the Methylphenidate (Ritalin) was a very mild medication and would stimulate the brain stem and help Matthew focus.

We gave into the schools pressure and took our son to a pediatrician that they recommended. His name was Dr. John Dorsey of Birmingham, Michigan. While visiting Dr. Dorsey with the schools recommendation for Methylphenidate (Ritalin) in hand, I noted that he seemed frustrated with the school. He asked us to remind the school that he was not a pharmacy.

I can only conclude from his comment that we were not the first parents sent to him by this school. Dr. John Dorsey officially diagnosed Matthew with ADHD. The test used for the diagnosis was a five minute pencil twirling trick, resulting in Matthew being diagnosed with ADHD.

As described in Chapter Two of this book, when Matthew was 14 years old he had a heart attack and died. The cause of death was assigned to his long-term use of Ritalin. From his autopsy it was discovered that he had suffered serious heart damage from the use of the drug. What lead to his being given an ADHD diagnosis, his drugging and eventual death was a threat from a social worker about Child Protective Services being brought to bear against the family.

Section IV

The Narrow Scope of Psychiatry

Chapter Seventeen

The Narrow Scope of Psychiatry

The fact is, psychiatry and psychology have not given us much better understanding of Man; indeed, they seem to have muddied our understanding and common sense with their own confusions. They are still very primitive subjects, based almost wholly on assumptions, theories and beliefs. Although many researches are routinely conducted in these fields and though they attempt to follow scientific methods, one will not find solid, scientific, natural laws that have been isolated by these efforts, like one will find in the physical sciences.

On the contrary, these fields are awash with the ebb and flow of pet theories and fads as to why people do what they do and became the way they are. These fields are also awash with theories and fads as to approaches to take to Man's problems in life.

In short, one is not likely to find statistics or evidence of things improving where psychiatrists and psychologists are playing a major role. This fact is evident in our prison system, mental hospitals, various social programs and in our nation's schools. A blatant example occurring over the past decade was the continually rising numbers of U.S. military service members committing suicide coincident with the continual rise in mental health professionals prescribing psychiatric drugs for the soldiers. Many of the soldiers committing suicide had not been in combat, but had been undergoing treatment by mental health personnel. Unfortunately, some of the drugs the soldiers were being given, such as antidepressants, can increase suicidal thinking and behavior. Furthermore, the drugs have sometimes been given to the soldiers in outlandish combinations, such as being given around a dozen or more different types all at once.

There are tremendous ironies connected with psychiatry. One can think psychiatrists and their drugs are supposed to make people saner and yet they can make them insane and suicidal. Because of the worsening state of affairs and increased suicides in the military, psychiatrists can request more funding from the government (taxpayers) to handle the suicide problem and they can get it. Then they increase the number of soldiers they drug. Then there are even greater numbers of suicides per year and the psychiatrists would ask for more money, and so it goes. This cycle, with its continually rising costs in deaths and money can go on for years. Witness that it already has.

Bluntly, psychiatrists today do not even have a rudimentary understanding of how the mind works.

They do not know how it is accomplished that you can read these symbols (written letters) and get what is being communicated.

They do not know how you can recall in detail your experience of having breakfast this morning: what you ate, where you sat, what you saw, the temperature of the room and what you were thinking about at the time.

They don't know how you can store all your memories in color, with motion and when they occurred, all in great detail, including your thoughts and decisions at the time. They don't have the faintest idea how all that data is stored, never mind elicited or reasoned with.

They don't know how you create new ideas that are not recordings, or how a composer hears a new melody in his mind, a painter creates an art work or a father conceives of a way to make his daughter have a joyous birthday or where Man's massive intelligence and ability to resolve problems comes from.

They may have an idea that some "chemical messengers" go from one brain neuron (nerve cell) to another, but how does that explain how you can recall all the different things you did yesterday or what your home was like when you were 5 years old? How does that explain your mind and all its recordings and complete memories of experiences, not to mention the person, the entity that is looking at the memories and choosing which ones to look at? Both the person, in making a decision, and his or her mind, can and do effect the transport of chemicals between neurons and their abundance. Amazingly, psychiatrists often ignore the person himself and his mind and remain preoccupied with the chemicals in the synapses (spaces between nerve cells).

152

The narrowness of psychiatric address to human behavior problems funnels the psychiatrist in the direction of chemical alteration as his main solution. If a child is having difficulty in school, a psychiatrist or psychologist is likely to assign a wrong cause for the difficulty and start to address it. It is very likely they will try to label the child with the title of a made-up disease. The psychiatrist may try to convince the child and his or her parents that the child has a defect in his brain and that he should be drugged for the defect with one or more drugs, such as methylphenidate or amphetamines. But he can't show the parent proof of the defect and the drugs may cause real defects in the child's brain, as well as stunting of the child's whole body, including his brain. Numerous other "side effects" are likely to ensue. This is mental "health" treatment today.

In past decades and centuries, even a few decades ago, Man did not drug children who were struggling in school or having trouble settling down in stifling classroom settings or who were bored stiff with certain classes and aspects of their education. Drugging children on a massive scale with amphetamines is a psychiatric solution to these difficulties in education, a very recent development in human history. Man successfully evolved and learned without this solution, until the last 40 years or so.

The massive drugging of children in Western society with amphetamines, antipsychotics, antidepressants and other psychiatric drugs is a very dangerous trend that is occurring today. It is dangerous because these drugs may physically damage children permanently, including their brains. Another reason it is dangerous is that many of the drugs circulating through our educational systems and households are extremely addictive. When children and grownups become addicted to amphetamines or other drugs, their personal ethics are likely to deteriorate and they will often be found doing things injurious to themselves, their families and society.

This trend needs to be halted and reversed for the sake of our present and future civilization. Our schoolchildren should not be treated as a psychiatric drug market and turned into people who will grow up thinking that psychiatric drugs are the solutions when one is faced with difficulties or challenges in life. Someone who faces challenges without a chemical crutch and succeeds comes to realize they are capable of doing it again and again.

In Conclusion

Our nation's children should not be viewed or treated as a massive drug market. They should be viewed and strengthened as those who will be responsible for our future civilization.

Parents need to understand how deceptive the diagnosing process is in psychiatry and the damage that psychiatric drugs can cause to their children. The chances are that if you start your child on an ADHD drug, the child's growth will be stunted for life, including the growth of his or her overall body and brain. Many other side effects will be caused. Yet the child's academic performance will not really be enhanced in the long term. It is likely that it may even be worsened. Realize that causing stunted body growth and numerous other damaging effects to a child's body from ADHD drugs is acceptable to most psychiatrists. They are not really in the "health" business; they are mostly in the drugging business.

Children need loving parents, a safe and sane environment, good nutrition and help with understanding things they don't understand, including difficult areas in their schoolwork. These factors are in the province of parental responsibility, not the psychiatrists'.

Sources

Section I   **Side Effects from ADHD Drugs No Child Would Want**

CHAPTER ONE: **PHYSICAL SIDE EFFECTS FROM ADHD DRUGS**

Nursing 87 Drug Handbook, "Cerebral Stimulants, Central Nervous System Drugs," section on methylphenidate hydrochloride, Springhouse Corporation, Springhouse, PA, 1987, p. 305.

Miranda Hitti, "ADHD Drug Cylert Discontinued," webmd.com, March 25, 2005.

Weiss et al. "Effects of long-term treatment of hyperactive children with methylphenidate," *Canadian Medical Association Journal,* Vol. 112, No.2, 1975, p. 164.

CHAPTER TWO: **ADHD DRUGS AND SHORTENING OF LIFE SPAN**

Sam's statement found in an article by Angela Hennessy "Adderall Can Really Fuck You Up," VICE Canada.

Associated Press, "FDA Won't Ban Drug for ADHD," *Washington Post,* Feb 11, 2005, p. A07.

Carl Sherman Ph.D., "The Adderall Ban in Canada," website ADDitude, April, 2005.

156

Associated Press, "Ritalin is blamed for teenager's death," *The Boston Globe,* April, 17, 2000.

Jon E. Doherty, "Ritalin's long-term effects questioned, Death of 14-year-old boy highlights concerns over popular drug," WorldNetDaily.com, May 8, 2000, p. 1, website ritalindeath. com

Dave Savini, "The highs and lows of Ritalin," msnbc.com, May 2, 2000, pp. 3-4.

Vicki Duncle, "Psychotropic Drugs and Failure to Warn," ritalindeath.com

Product information sheet for Adderall, Shire US, Inc., 2011.

CHAPTER THREE: **STUNTED BODY GROWTH FROM TAKING AHDH DRUGS**

Weiss et al. "Effect of long-term treatment of hyperactive children with methylphenidate," *Canadian Medical Association Journal,* Vol. 112, No. 2, 1975, p. 164.

Megan C. Lisska and Scott A. Rivkees, Department of Pediatrics of the Yale University School of Medicine, "Daily Methylphenidate Use Slows the Growth of Children: A Community Based Study," *Journal of Pediatric Endocrinology & Metabolism,* Vol. 16, 2003, pp. 711-718.

A. Poulton and C.T. Cowell, Department of Paediatrics, Nepean Hospital, Penrith and Institute of Paediatric Endocrinology, Children's Hospital at Westmead, New South Wales, Australia, "Slowing of growth in height and weight on stimulants: A characteristic pattern," *Journal of Paediatrics and Child Health*, Vol. 39, 2003, pp. 180-185.

Jared Owens, "Ritalin linked to growth delays in adolescent boys," *The Australian*, Jan. 22, 2013.

CHAPTER FOUR: EVIDENCE OF BRAIN DAMAGE
                 AND BRAIN SHRINKAGE FROM
                 ADHD DRUGS

Sandra Blakeslee, "This Is Your Brain on Meth: A 'Forest Fire' of Damage," *The New York Times*, July 20, 2004.

Fred A. Baughman, Jr. M.D., "The Totality of the ADD/ADHD Fraud," 1998.

F. Xavier Castellanos, M.D. et al., "Quantitative Brain Magnetic Imaging in Attention-Deficit Hyperactivity Disorder," *Archives of General Psychiatry*, Vol. 53, July 1996, pp. 607-616.

P.A. Filipek, M.D. et al., "Volumetric MRI analysis comparing subjects having attention-deficit hyperactivity disorder with normal controls," *Neurology*, Vol. 48, No. 3, March 1997, pp. 589-601.

Jonathan Leo and David Cohen, "Broken Brains or Flawed Studies, A Critical Review of ADHD Neuroimaging Research," *The Journal of Mind and Behavior*, Vol. 24, Winter 2003.

National Institute of Mental Health press release, "Brain Shrinkage in ADHD Not Caused by Medications," Oct. 8, 2002.

Jonathan Leo and David Cohen, "An Update on ADHD Neuroimaging Research," *The Journal of Mind and Behavior*, Vol. 25, No. 2, Spring 2004, pp. 161-166.

Fred A. Baughman, M.D., "The 'Chemical Imbalance' Lie Dooms Informed Consent," Testimony of Fred A.

Baughman, M.D., to the March 23, 2006 [FDA] meeting of the Psychopharmacologic Drugs Advisory Committee.

Henry A. Nasrallah M.D. et al., "Cortical Atrophy in Young Adults With a History of Hyperactivity in Childhood," *Psychiatry Research,* Vol. 17, 1986, pp. 241-246.

Gene-Jack Wang et al., "Methylphenidate Decreases Regional Cerebral Blood Flow in Normal Human Subjects," *Life Sciences, Including Pharmacology Letters,* Vol. 54, Nov. 9, 1994, pp. 144-146.

Deborah Kotz, "Pulling an all-nighter could damage brain, study suggests," *boston.com,* Jan. 2, 2014.

CHAPTER FIVE: **DAMAGING PSYCHOLOGICAL EFFECTS FROM BEING DIAGNOSED AND DRUGGED FOR ADHD**

Richard Scarnati, D.O., "An Outline of the Hazardous Effects of Ritalin (Methlphenidate)," *The International Journal of the Addictions,* Vol. 21, 1986, pp. 837-841.

Diagnostic and Statistical Manual of Mental Disorders, Third Edition, Revised, American Psychiatric Association, Washington, DC., 1987, p. 175.

Robert Whitacker and Delores Kong, "Doing Harm: Research on the Mentally Ill, Testing takes human toll," *Boston Sunday Globe,* Nov. 15, 1998, p. A32.

Robert Whitacker and Delores Kong, "Doing Harm: Research on the Mentally Ill," the full series of articles, *The Boston Globe,* Nov 15, 16 ,17 ,18, 1998.

Product information sheet for Ritalin, CIBA Pharmaceutical Company, Division of CIBA-Geigy Corporation, Summit, N.J., 1985.

Katy Corneel and David S. Kiffer, "Matthew's defense may end today," *The Patriot Ledger,* Quincy, MA, March 7, 1988, pp. 1, 12.

Ed Hayward, "Son charged in family slayings: Ritalin use probed in teen's alleged rampage," *Boston Herald,* Oct. 12, 1993, pp. 1, 6.

Kelly Patricia O'Meara, "Doping Kids," *Insight Magazine,* Vol. 15, No. 24, June 28, 1999, insight magazine.com, p. 1.

CHAPTER SIX: **DRUG ADDICTION FROM TAKING RITALIN, AMPHETAMINES AND COCAINE AND WHY THEY ARE CATEGORIZED TOGETHER**

http://www.deadiversion.usdoj.gov/schedules/, Lists of Scheduling Actions/Controlled Substances.

Everett Ellinwood and M. Marlyne Kilbey, "Stimulant Abuse in Man: The Use of Animal Models to Assess and Predict Human Toxicity," *Predicting Dependence Liability of Stimulant and Depressant Drugs,* University Park Press, Baltimore, MD., 1977, p. 83.

Diagnostic and Statistical Manual of Mental Disorders, Third Edition, Revised, American Psychiatric Association, Washington, DC., 1987, p. 175.

Kenneth Whyte et al., "A prescribed urban nightmare: How two obscure, legal drugs unleashed a wave of crime in the streets," *Western Report,* Vol. 2, No. 2, Feb. 2, 1987, p. 38.

Richard Chacon, "On campus, Ritalin getting attention as a good 'buzz'," *The Boston Globe*, Feb. 12, 1998, p. A10.

Sabrina Tavernise, "New Sign of Stimulants' Toll on Young," *The New York Times*, Aug. 8, 2013.

Dr. Ronald Ricker and Dr. Venus Nicolino, "Adderall: The Most Abused Prescription Drug in America," huffingtonpost. com, June 21, 2010. CGuy, comment posted to the mentioned article, July 1, 2010.

Dan Harris and Lana Zak, "Supermom's Secret Addiction: Stepping Out of Adderall's Shadow," ABC News, June 26, 2012.

Student, 18 year old from Sarasota Florida, posted statement about "Study Drugs," on NYTimes.com, June 6, 2012.

Alan Schwarz, "Drowned in a Stream of Prescriptions,"*The New York Times*, Feb. 2, 2013.

Section II   **The Diagnosis of ADHD By Opinion, Not Scientific or Medical Testing**

CHAPTER SEVEN: PSYCHIATRY'S DIAGNOSTIC AND STATISTICAL MANUAL OF MENTAL DISORDERS AND THE ADHD DIAGNOSIS

Diagnostic and Statistical Manual of Mental Disorders, Version 4, American Psychiatric Association, Washington, D.C.

Herb Kutchins and Stuart A. Kirk, *Making Us Crazy*, The Free Press, New York, 1997, pp. 52-53, 55-99.

Fred A. Baughman, Jr., M.D., "Immunize Your Child Against Attention Deficit Disorder (ADD)," http://www.whale.to/a/baughman1.html

Centers for Disease Control and Prevention (website), "Attention-Deficit/Hyperactivity Disorder (ADHD), Data & Statistics."

"ADHD, Symptoms and Diagnosis," Centers for Disease Control and Prevention (CDC). 2014.

CHAPTER EIGHT: THE YOUNGER STUDENTS IN CLASSROOMS TEND TO BE DIAGNOSED ADHD CONSIDERABLY MORE THAN THE OLDER ONES

Anahad O'Connor, "Younger Students More Likely to Get A.D.H.D. Drugs," *The Well* (blog), Nov 20, 2012.

Rick Nauert, Ph.D., "Youngest Kids in Class Get More ADHD Diagnoses, Drugs," psychcentral.com, Mar. 6, 2012.

"Nearly 1 million children potentially misdiagnosed with ADHD, study finds," MSU News, Aug 17, 2010.

CHAPTER NINE: BOYHOOD CHARACTERISTICS HAVE BEEN TURNED INTO SYMPTOMS OF IMAGINED ADHD

E. Mark Mahone, Ph.D., "Neuropsychiatric Differences Between Boys and Girls with ADHD," PsychiatricTimes.Com, Oct. 3, 2012.

Jeanie Russell, "The Pill That Teachers Push," *Good Housekeeping,* Dec. 1996.

Centers for Disease Control and Prevention (website), "Attention Deficit/Hyperactivity Disorder (ADHD) Data and Statistics" in the United States, from survey conducted in 2011.

Alan Schwarz and Sarah Cohen, "A.D.H.D. Seen in 11% of U.S. Children as Diagnoses Rise," *New York Times,* Mar. 31, 2013.

CHAPTER TEN: PSYCHIATRY'S DIAGNOSTIC MANUAL AND THEIR INSINUATION INTO THE FIELD OF MEDICINE

Diagnostic and Statistical Manual of Mental Disorders, Version Number 4, American Psychiatric Association, Washington, D.C.

Loren R. Mosher, M.D., Letter of Resignation from the American Psychiatric Association (APA), Dec. 4, 1998.

Felicity Berringer, from the *New York Times* News Service, "Soviet Psychiatry Still Under a Cloud," *Chicago Tribune*, Oct. 21, 1987.

Paul Quinn-Judge, "Gorbachev reinforces reform image by freeing dissidents," *The Christian Science Monitor*, Feb. 9, 1987.

Section III **Influences Behind the Drugging of Children for ADHD**

CHAPTER ELEVEN: **PEOPLE CAN THINK ADHD DRUGS WILL IMPROVE A CHILD'S ACADEMIC PERFORMANCE**

L. Alan Sroufe, "Ritalin Gone Wrong," *The New York Times*, Jan. 28, 2012.

Alan Schwarz, "Risky Rise of the Good-Grade Pill," *The New York Times*, June 9, 2012.

Linda Charles and Richard Schain, "A Four-Year Follow-up Study of the Effects of Methylphenidate on the Behavior and Academic Achievement of Hyperactive Children," *Journal of Abnormal Child Psychology*, Vol. 9, No. 4, December 1981, p. 504.

Michael P. Aman, Ph.D., and John S. Werry, M.D., "Methylphenidate and Diazapam in Severe Reading

Retardation," *Journal of the American Academy of Child Psychology*, Vol. 21, No. 1, 1982, p. 36.

Kenneth D. Gadow, Ph.D., "Effects of Stimulant Drugs on Academic Performance in Hyperactive and Learning Disabled Children," *Journal of Learning Disabilities*, Vol. 16, No. 5, May, 1983, p. 291.

Teodoro Ayllon, Dale Layman and Henry J. Kandel, "A Behavioral-Educational Alternative to Drug Control of Hyperactive Children," *Journal of Applied Behavior Analysis*, Vol. 8, No. 2, Summer 1975, p. 144.

Rachel Gittelman, Donald Klein and Ingrid Feingold, "Effects of Methylphenidate in Combination with Reading Remediation," *Journal of Child Psychology and Psychiatry*, Vol. 24, No. 2, April 1983, p. 210.

Russell A. Barkley, Ph.D., Charles E. Cunningham, Ph.D., "Do Stimulant Drugs Improve the Academic Performance of Hyperkinetic Children?: A Review of Outcome Studies," *Clinical Pediatrics*, Vol. 17, January, 1978, p. 90.

Herbert E. Rie, Ph.D. et al., "Effects of Ritalin on Underachieving Children," *American Journal of Orthopsychiatry*, Vol. 46, No. 2, April 1976, p. 320.

Gerald Coles, *The Learning Mystique, A Critical Look at "Learning Disabilities,"* Pantheon Books, New York, 1987, p. 94.

Katherine Sharpe, "Medication: The smart-pill oversell, Evidence is mounting that medication for ADHD doesn't make a lasting difference to schoolwork or achievement," *Nature*, Feb 12, 2014.

CHAPTER TWELVE: DIAGNOSING AND DRUGGING
CHILDREN FOR ADHD IS
PROFITABLE

Alan Schwarz, "The Selling of Attention Deficit Disorder," *The New York Times*, Dec. 14, 2013.

CHAPTER THIRTEEN: DRUG COMPANIES REWARD
PSYCHIATRISTS AND DOCTORS
WHO PRESCRIBE AND
PROMOTE THEIR DRUGS

Benedict Carey and Gardiner Harris, "Psychiatric Group Faces Scrutiny over Drug Industry Ties," *The New York Times*, July 12, 2008.

Emily Ramshaw and Ryan Murphy, "Payments to Doctors by Pharmaceutical Companies Raise Issues of Conflicts," *The New York Times*, November 24, 2011.

Gardiner Harris and Benedict Carey, "Researchers Fail to Report Full Drug Pay," *The New York Times*, June 8, 2008.

Alan Schwarz, "The Selling of Attention Deficit Disorder," *The New York Times*, Dec. 14, 2013.

Cathleen Pearson, "Antipsychotics Prescribed To Treat ADHD In More Children And Teens, New Study Finds," huffingtonpost.com, August 9, 2012.

David Muzina, M.D., "Turning Attention to ADHD: U.S. Medication Trends for Attention Deficit Hyperactivity Disorder," lab.express-scripts.com, Mar. 17, 2014.

Gardiner Harris, "Popular Drugs for Dementia Tied to Deaths," *The New York Times*, April 12, 2005.

Joe Parks, M.D. et al., "Morbidity and Mortality in People with Serious Mental Illness," Report for the National Association of State Mental Health Program Directors, Oct. 2006.

Claudia Dreifus, "A Conversation With Nancy C. Andreasen," *The New York Times*, Sept. 16, 2008.

Beng-Choon Ho, MRCPsych; Nancy C. Andreasen, M.D., Ph.D; et al., "Long-term Antipsychotic Treatment and Brain Volumes: A Longitudinal Study of First-Episode Schizophrenia," (Abstract), *Archives of General Psychiatry*, February 7, 2011.

Tracy Weber and Charles Ornstein, "Dollars for Docs Mints a Millionaire," ProPublica.org, Mar. 11, 2013.

E. Haavi Morreim, "Prescribing Under the Influence," excerpted from a presentation she made for the Markkula Ethics Center Lecture Series at Santa Clara University.

Shantanu Agrawal, M.D., Niall Brennan, M.P.P., and Peter Budetti, M.D., J.D., "The Sunshine Act - Effects on Physicians," *New England Journal of Medicine*, 2013; 368; 2054-2057, May 30, 2013.

Chapter Fourteen:

U.S. Government Program Rewards Parents for Drugging Their Children

Patricia Wen, "Pathologist: Rebecca Riley died of pneumonia, toxic level of drugs," boston.com, Jan. 28, 2010.

Patricia Wen, "Psychiatrist admits she approved higher drug dosage in Riley trail," boston.com, January 25, 2010.

Scott Allen, "Backlash on bipolar diagnoses in children," boston.com, June 17, 2007.

Lawrence Diller, "Misguided Standards of Care," *The Boston Globe*, June 19, 2007.

Denise Lavoie, "Father Seeks New Trial in Daughter's 2006 Overdose Death," boston.cbslocal.com, Nov. 28, 2013.

Patricia Wen, "A legacy of unintended side effects," *The Boston Globe*, December 12-14, 2010.

CHAPTER FIFTEEN: **SCHOOLS HAVE BEEN TURNED INTO A MAIN MARKETING TOOL FOR THE PSYCHIATRIC CHILD-DRUGGING INDUSTRY**

Education for All Handicapped Children Act of 1975, Subchapter 1, General Provisions, Section 1401, Definitions (a), (1).

For SAT scores, Educational Testing Services, Princeton N.J.

For full text of Elementary and Secondary Education Act of 1965, google "original text of 1965 esea act"

Diagnostic and Statistical Manual of Mental Disorders, all editions, American Psychiatric Association, Washington, D.C.

Education Week, April 24, 1984, quoted by Samuel L. Blumenfeld, *NEA, Trojan Horse in American Education,* The Paradigm Company, Boise, Idaho, 1984, p.128.

Joseph P. Shapiro et al., "Separate and Unequal," *U.S. News and World Report*, Dec. 13, 1993, pp. 47-48.

For data on "Individuals with Disabilities Act (IDEA)", google idea.ed.gov

For statistics on male and female prescriptions of ADHD drugs, google Centers for Disease Control (CDC).

The Editorial Board, "Worry Over Attention Deficit Cases," *The New York Times*, April 9, 2013.

CHAPTER SIXTEEN:	**PARENTS CAN BE THREATENED WITH HAVING THEIR CHILDREN TAKEN AWAY IF THEY *DON'T* DRUG THEM**

The Smith Family, Death from Ritalin, The Truth Behind ADHD (website). (This website can also be reached at Ritalindeath.com)

Section IV   The Narrow Scope of Psychiatry

CHAPTER SEVENTEEN:

THE NARROW SCOPE OF PSYCHIATRY

Dozens of cases of American soldiers committing suicide while taking antidepressants (and other psychiatric drugs) can be found at the website http://ssristories.org/category/ occupation/military/. The site also provides documentation for each of its cases.

CPSIA information can be obtained at www.ICGtesting.com
Printed in the USA
BVOW11s1817250615

406216BV00011B/40/P